Cat's Claw

HEALING VINE
OF PERU

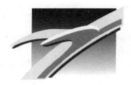

KENNETH
JONES

Sylvan Press
Seattle, Washington

Sylvan Press
1202 East Pike Street, Suite 746
Seattle, Washington 98122

Disclaimer: Individuals seeking relief from a health condition should seek the advice of a qualified health practitioner. The information in this book cannot and is not intended to replace the skills of a professional.

Cover and page design by Rich Rawling, Cortex Consultants Inc.

ISBN: 0-9625638-3-8

Printed in Hong Kong

Acknowledgments

There are many to whom I am ever grateful for aiding me in the task of writing this book. Thanks are especially due to Sylvan and the cats; Jeff Chilton for keeping the project on track and for excellent organizational input; Patricia Wolfe for her excellent editorial attention to so many critical details; and to Fred Katz for superb translations of Spanish documents and careful editorial work which allowed this book to be completed on time without compromising the breadth of the information at hand. For their research assistance and warm hospitality, I am ever grateful to Gladys Reverditto and family; Guisella Tesoro Brell and family; The Association for the Conservation of the Patrimony of Cutivireni (ACPC); and my guides in Peru, who have chosen to remain anonymous.

Contents

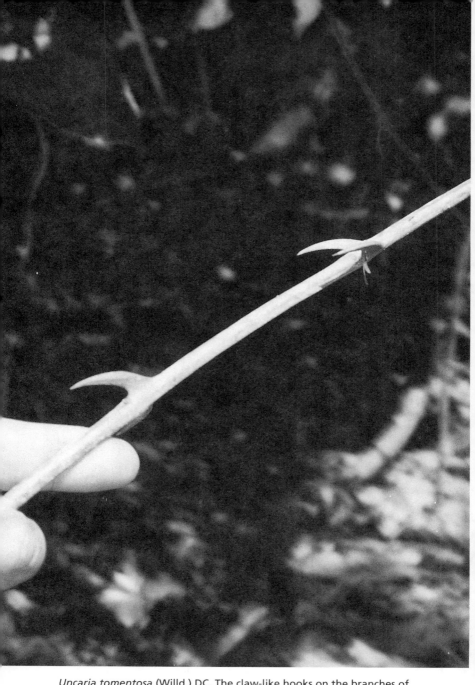

Uncaria tomentosa (Willd.) DC. The claw-like hooks on the branches of the vine resulted in the common name *uña de gato* or "cat's claw."

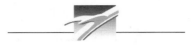

Introduction

In the forests of Peru there are two massive woody vines or lianas, both known as "uña de gato," a Spanish name meaning "cat's claw." They are distinct species of *Uncaria* which received their Spanish common name in reference to the curved back hooks (*uncus*) that occur in pairs on either side of the stem at the leaf junctions. Catching the branches of other plants, these hooks allow the vines to suspend their weight as they grow up from the darkness of the jungle floor towards the sunlight.

In Geneva, in May 1994, the World Health Organization sponsored the First International Conference on Uña de Gato where the vine received official recognition as a medicinal plant.[1,2] As one writer has already pointed out, it is fair to say that since the 17th century when the bark of "quina-quina" trees (*Cinchona*) became the treatment of choice for malaria and later gave the world the anti-malarial drug quinine, no plant from the Peruvian forests has prompted such world attention.[3] It is perhaps significant that the two plants, cat's claw (*Uncaria*) and quina-quina (*Cinchona*), are members of the same plant family, Rubiaceae.

I first learned of "cat's thorn" from researchers in Germany in 1984, during my studies of another South American medicinal plant—pau d'arco (*Tabebuia* species). By 1994, the vine had become a subject of great interest in the West, so I began to collect the facts about this folk medicine. Eventually, I retraced the history of cat's claw from the natural pharmacy of the Peruvian Indians to the laboratories of Europe. My quest for factual information culminated in this book. Apart from providing substantive information on the application and activities of cat's claw, this book is intended to foster ecological respect for the vine and for those to whom we are rightly indebted for medical knowledge of cat's claw in the first place—the Indians of Peru and those humble enough to listen to their ways.

Kenneth Jones,
December 1995.

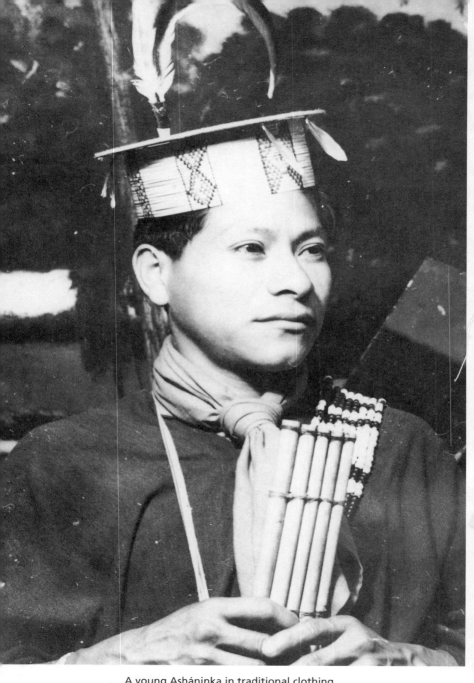

A young Asháninka in traditional clothing.

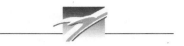

I.

Adventurers and Indians

Early Explorers

All but forgotten for the past 20 years, one of the first Europeans to experiment with cat's claw was a young Bavarian schoolteacher named Arturo Brell. His experience with the medicinal vine resurfaced in Peru in April 1995. Writing for the Lima newspaper *El Mundo*, Jose Luis Hidalgo learned that in 1964 Brell had collaborated on recording native uses of the vine with an American named Eugene Whitworth, a professor from Great Western University in San Francisco, California. Although Brell was already well-acquainted with cat's claw, together they made an expedition to collect medicinal plants from several tribes in Peru, among them the Shipibo and Asháninka Indians. Professor Whitworth returned to California with 22 plant samples, including the vine the Indians called *zavenna rozza* or *uña de gato*. A year later, in Germany, Brell recounted his interest in the vine in an interview for a German magazine. Hidalgo also learned that during his visit to Germany, Brell had given an extract of the vine to a cousin who had been diagnosed with breast cancer. Her recovery was complete and her doctors were astounded.[4]

In the early 1930s, Brell realized a childhood ambition with an opportunity to work in the land of the Incas and to live among the Indians. His immigration to Peru was arranged by a priest from Pozuzo, the site of a German community in the Province of Chanchamayo, located 131 miles east of Lima. Brell's job was to set up a school to teach the Indians the ways of modern European society. However, what he learned from the Indians proved to be of far greater value.[4]

In the Valley of Entaz, where Brell grew coffee and lived and worked with the Indians, he noticed that cancer didn't seem to afflict the natives, even though they were constantly subjected to the hazards of burnt grease, resins, and smoke and tars from their cooking and heating fires. Applying insights gleaned from his training in biology in Munich, Brell surmised that the teas in their diet were acting as protectants against carcinogens. The mechanism, he reasoned, would most likely be an interaction of the teas with the immune system.[4]

Among the plants consumed by the Indians was a woody vine with a name that sounded like "zavenna rozza." The same plant was known by the Spanish name "uña de gato" and the inner bark was boiled to make a tea. Among other uses, it was used by the Indian women as a contraceptive. Brell had used the vine himself and found it improved his skin, made his hair grow faster, and eliminated the painful rheumatism from which he had suffered for years.[4]

Arturo Brell passed away in Lima, in 1978, at the age of 74. In his belongings were hundreds of testimonial letters from people expressing their gratitude for the benefits they experienced through the botanical formulas Brell formulated with cat's claw.[1] These facts left me wondering whatever had happened to Brell's work. It was a piece of history that I grew determined to follow. Eventually, after a year collecting information on cat's claw, I decided to travel to Peru to uncover the missing history of Brell.

While preparing for Peru, I was lucky enough to find the same Professor Eugene Whitworth alive and well and living in San Francisco. Would he remember Arturo Brell and a vine used by the Indians? We were about to talk about an episode in his life going back 30 years. In answer to my question, he laughed and explained how his time with Brell was an experience that even someone as old as he would never forget.[5]

Cat's claw was boiled and the brew produced was rich in alkaloids.

It all began in the early 1960s. Along with a medical officer named Claude Yates, he and a party of five had been given a grant to travel to Peru to record native dances before they became another item on the already growing list of lost arts. The trip was expected to be one big adventure holiday, or so he thought. Before leaving he received a call from a man who claimed the natives of Peru had cures for all kinds of diseases, even cancer. Out of simple curiosity, Whitworth contacted a doctor in Lima who would direct him to a guide to help him interview Indians about dances and cures. His journey eventually led to Brell and the two of them set out on various expeditions to remote areas of Peru.[5]

Whitworth had fond memories of his time with Brell: the many wondrous plants they examined; the secrets of their uses received from the shamans; and the colorful tribes they stopped to consult along the rivers. In one instance, Whitworth related his amazement at being shown a tree that from one side was used to provide bark for a tea to ensure a woman's fertility, but from the other side served to prevent pregnancy for as long as three years.[5]

He remembered that Brell had sent samples of cat's claw to botanists in Europe who had identified the vine. Cat's claw was boiled and the brew produced was rich in alkaloids which tended to lose their strength (or pH) unless stabilized. To accomplish this, Brell added some leaf material from another plant and eventually developed an herbal formula. Doctors from all over the world requested the extract, some from as far away as Romania, India, and England. Whitworth still had one of the old bottles with the ingredients on the label. Doubting the label contained the real recipe, I suggested he keep it from prying eyes; phony formulas are the last thing anyone needs if they are seriously ill,[5] and today there are plenty of unscrupulous profiteers who would eagerly exploit such an obvious opportunity.

Now Whitworth insisted that I make him a promise. During my investigations in Peru, I had to at least try to find Brell's little clinic. It was somewhere near San Ramón, 124 miles northeast of Lima. Whitworth had never forgotten the day Brell had written to inform him of the newly established "Whitworth Cancer Research Center." In what Whitworth described as typical Brell humor, Brell joked about how well-equipped the Center was — it had a heliport, a donkey port, and a canoe port.[5] While I doubted the clinic would even be standing today, I made the promise to try to locate it.

Whitworth went on to recall how the doctor in Lima who had arranged to find a guide for the expedition had been delighted to learn of their subsequent success. Whitworth was certain that Brell had eventually managed to obtain permission from the authorities in Peru to conduct a clinical study. He explained that, on his own, Brell had already compared the outcomes of 100 terminal cancer patients, who used the extract, to a control group of cancer patients who hadn't. Brell then waited the full five years to determine if the treatment was successful or if the remissions were only temporary. Whitworth recalled that when all the patients had been checked, 64 out of the 100 who had received the extract were still alive and in good health. I reminded him how today a rate of cancer remission that high would be considered good by any standards, but how before the results would ever be accepted, such a study would have to be repeated in more controlled settings.[5]

Whitworth continued his recollections, explaining how he had waited patiently for Brell's results in hopes of having some-

thing substantial to present to scientists in the U.S. But no one
wanted to look at it. Instead, he was told to stop making such a
fool of himself. He finally gave up and the work of Brell has
been languishing ever since.[5]

He called the vine "saventaro," an Asháninka name meaning powerful (antearo) plant (saveshi).

Despite the sketchiness of Professor Whitworth's recollections, the saga of Brell hadn't lost any of its allure. If anything,
it had become that much more intriguing. I made plans to do
some research of my own in Peru, for as Whitworth lamented,
his notes and the many letters Brell had written on his progress
with the remedy were now so aged they were hopelessly illegi-
ble. Whitworth and I concluded our conversation with plans to
discuss the subject of Arturo Brell again when I returned from
my investigations in Peru.

During the course of my research in preparation for Peru, the
name of another early explorer of cat's claw came to my attention with increasing frequency. This was Klaus Keplinger, a
journalist and self-taught ethnologist from Innsbruck, Austria
who had been investigating the activity of the vine for the last
20 years.[6,7] Although he began his research after Brell,[8,9]
Keplinger was responsible for organizing the first definitive
studies, all at great personal expense.

Keplinger began seriously looking into cat's claw several
years after cancer had claimed the life of a close friend and
former climbing companion. In 1959, they scaled mountains in
the Cordillera Blanca,[10,11] a stunning range located in the
northern part of Peru.[12] Keplinger was led to cat's claw by the
granddaughter of a Peruvian man who had nearly died from
advanced-stage lung cancer in 1968.[13] In response to his
friend's untimely demise, Keplinger vowed to investigate the

vine in the hope of discovering something that might compensate for his friend's death. He had been seriously interested in ethnobotany for many years and wanted to write an in-depth article on the vine for European publication. However, as the pace of his research accelerated, his focus shifted dramatically from wanting to write about cat's claw to actually bringing it to a university where it could be thoroughly investigated.[10]

Arriving in Peru to begin his research, Keplinger visited the Peruvian man who had come close to dying from lung cancer. He was a sawmill owner named Luis Oscar Schuler.[14,15] The story of how this man had been treated with a tea made from a vine had reached Keplinger through Schuler's granddaughter who, at the time, was attending university in Innsbruck.[16] Schuler lived in the same area as Brell, in a region of central Peru known as the Chanchamayo Valley and had taken an extract of cat's claw and other herbs provided by Brell who was known locally as an expert on Peruvian medicinal plants.[14,15] Brell, who knew the uses of at least 300 different herbs, was using both species of cat's claw and something called "cebollera hembra," which was possibly some species of *Allium*. At the time, Schuler was also receiving cobalt treatments, but chose to keep his herbal self-medication secret from his doctors.[15]

Around the same time Mr. Schuler had begun taking Brell's extract, his son Oscar was given the root of cat's claw to boil in order to make a curative tea for his father. While supervising the work on a new road to Puerto Bermúdez, Oscar was approached by his house maid who inquired about his father's condition. When Oscar confided he expected his father would soon die, she offered to call upon the services of her father, an Asháninka shaman. The shaman, who prescribed the root for both contraceptive purposes as well as the treatment of tumors, instructed Oscar in the preparation and dosage of the root tea. He called the vine "saventaro," an Asháninka name meaning powerful (antearo) plant (saveshi).[17]

At the time, Schuler was so sick that he could barely breathe and had to sleep sitting up. When his appetite dropped off and his terrible pains, coughing, and expelling blood went on unabated, his family realized he was close to death. Two months and ten cobalt treatments later, his condition had improved so dramatically that his doctor was at a complete loss to explain the recovery. He had more or less written him off and expected little more from the cobalt treatments than a temporary prolongation of life. In another two years, Mr. Schuler was completely recovered and in 1974, six years after the remission of his lung cancer, one reporter found him, at the age of 82, still smoking his pipe and laboring away in his sawmill as if nothing had happened.[15] Schuler died at the age of 91. His case became famous in Peru and abroad and to this day continues to focus attention on the vine and its potential benefits.[3]

The shaman, who showed him the vine, carefully selected only one type.

During the period of 1979-1981, Keplinger traveled to central Peru, to the Province of Oxapampa. At the German settlement of Pozuzu, he collected specimens of cat's claw. Leaving nothing to chance, he employed the expert help of Dr. Herwig Teppner, Head of the Institute of Systematic Botany of the University of Graz, Austria, who made certain of the identity of the vine. It was *Uncaria tomentosa* (Willd.) DC.[18]

The research that followed was unrelenting and eventually encompassed some uses of the whole root and certain constituents, such as alkaloids that potentiate the immune system.[19] Keplinger brought the tea and extract of cat's claw to the people of Austria and Germany where, today, various preparations are stocked by the local pharmacies,[10] but only for prescription and when all other medications have proven unsatisfactory.[7]

For activity studies of the vine, Keplinger gathered the root at a location east of the Andes in the mountains near the rivers

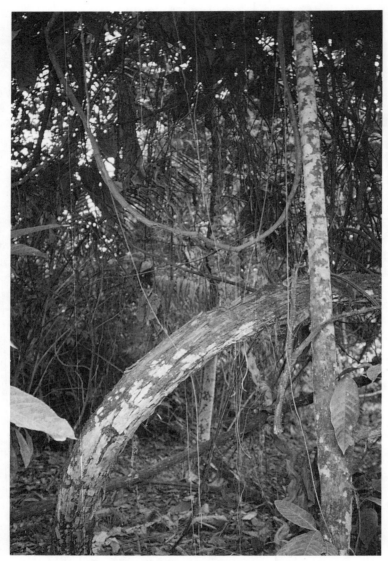

K. Jones, 1995

The curving base of a massive 90-foot cat's claw (*Uncaria tomentosa* (Willd.) DC) in the Chanchamayo Valley, Peru.

Perené and Chanchamayo at 1640 to 3937 feet above sea level.[19] The area is noted for its rainy and rugged forest, commonly known as the Ceja de la Montaña.[20] The shaman, who showed him the vine, carefully selected only one type. Eventually, the subtlety of the information being conveyed made it apparent to Keplinger that if he were to continue his field work with the Asháninka, he would have no choice but to learn their language. In his pursuit of their knowledge, Keplinger's interests grew beyond medicinal plants of the Asháninka and came to include them as a people. Since then his study of the Asháninka has been ongoing,[17] and his research to uncover an ancient written language of the Asháninka[21,22] and to record their folklore[23] reveal his genuine commitment to the preservation of their culture.

Traditional Records

An authority on the medicinal plants of Peru, Dr. Fernando Cabieses of the Peruvian Ministry of Health, had found *Uncaria* missing from the most important and even the oldest books on Peruvian medicinal plants,[3] and I was curious as to why. The article by Hidalgo in the Lima newspaper had mentioned use of the vine as a contraceptive.[4] That immediately implied that the vine, as part of the women's medicine, could have been largely kept from men which would include most ethnobotanists and explorers.[24] Or was it that the Indians who best knew its uses were, for a long time, too dangerous to approach? Such a description certainly fit the reputation of the Asháninka,[25] one of the main tribes that Brell and Whitworth had interviewed.[5] Yet, I couldn't rule out the possibility that the absence of cat's claw from the Peruvian records was simply attributable to its use being a jealously guarded secret of the shamans that few outsiders were ever privileged to learn.

Where they can be found, records of cat's claw's uses by the Indians of Peru are recent.[26] In *Witch Doctor's Apprentice* (Citadel Press, 1990), the famous American ethnobotanist Nicole Maxwell[27] wrote about people she had met during her long expeditions in Peru, who had successfully used the vine. They even treated difficult diseases, such as cancer, arthritis, and diabetes. She learned that another ethnobotanist working in Peru had found that among members of the Urarina tribe there were cases of cat's claw "curing tumors." In her own experience, when combined with antibiotics, the tea seemed to help her make a speedy recovery from surgery. She also noted that black hairs were appearing among her white ones—a side-effect of cat's claw she had been warned about beforehand.[28]

During a chance meeting over lunch in Iquitos, a middle-aged man at her table related that if it hadn't been for cat's claw he would have been dead from cancer years ago. Maxwell, who received medical training in the U.S., found her curiosity stirred and decided to examine his records from the Hospital del Empleado in Lima. He hadn't been exaggerating. Nine specialists attended the man and found generalized septicemia, severe cystitis, and a blood count that registered ten percent cancer cells. He might have received treatment, but the doctors had ordered him to leave; they were about to go on strike.[28]

Maxwell explained that when friends who knew herbal medicine came to the man's rescue, they were warned it would be very unusual for a patient in such an advanced stage of cancer to live another 10 days. Undeterred, they took him to their home where he was immediately given the sap of a tree called "sangre de grado" (*Croton lechleri*)—a few drops in water 'to heal the blood'—"chanca piedra" (*Phyllanthus niruri*) to treat his urinary tract infection, and the major herb in the prescription, cat's claw (*Uncaria tomentosa*). He went on to tell her about how he drank cat's claw all day, "every day." It was grated from the dried plant (20 grams) and boiled in one liter of water. After 14 days he got out of bed. Two weeks later, he strolled over to the hospital where he took immense pleasure in amazing his doctors. Maxwell learned that soon after he was well enough to return to work in Iquitos where he taught Spanish dance and ballet.[28]

Uña de Gato

There are many plants with the common name "uña de gato" which are not to be confused with the two species of *Uncaria* known as uña de gato in Peru: *Uncaria guianensis* (Aublet) Gmelin, and *Uncaria tomentosa* (Willdenow ex Roemer & Schultes) De Candolle.[26] At first glance, the two vines don't look much different until you see that in *U. guianensis* the hooks curve inward, whereas in *U. tomentosa* they protrude sharply. Another distinguishing characteristic is found in the leaves of the two species. The leaves of *guianensis* are narrower and shinier compared to those of *tomentosa,* which develop a dull appearance as they get older.[29] An easier method of distinguishing the two species is to count the numbers of lateral veins in the leaves. Whereas the leaves of *U. tomentosa* have eight to ten pairs of lateral veins, the leaves of *U. guianensis* may have six to seven alternating pairs.[30]

Traditional uses of these plants are practically identical. At the far northwestern corner of Peru in the Province of Huancabamba, the bark of cat's claw (*U. guianensis*) is used by the shamans of Piura to treat tumors, inflammations, rheumatism and gastric ulcers. In addition, the bark decoction is drunk as a contraceptive. They call the vine "garabato," meaning pothook.[31] This same plant is a source of potable water which is naturally stored in the center of the vine[26]—a fact that may explain the vine's listing among the edible plants of the world.[32] Other common names in Peru include "toroñ" (Yanesha Indian), and "aun huasca."[30]

In Colombia, the Boras Indians have used *Uncaria guianensis* to treat gonorrhea[33] while a different tribe, living in the region of Río Apaporis, have used the vine to prepare a tea for treating dysentery.[34] The same use is found in Suriname in northeast South America, where the leaves of "parrot's claw" (popokainangra) are prepared as an extract to treat dysentery and intestinal affections in young children. The leaves are also dried

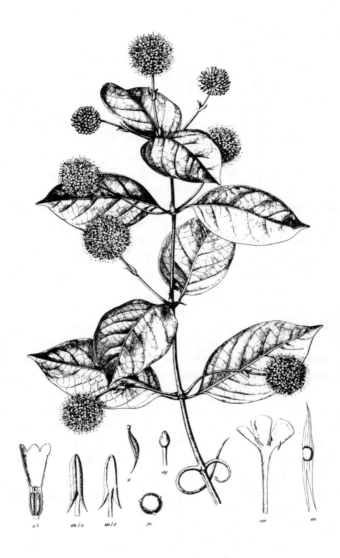

Uncaria guianensis (Aubl.) Gmel.

From Carlos F.P. De Martius and Augustus G. Eichler, *Flora Brasiliensis*, 1888-1889, vol. 6, part 6. (Weinheim, Germany: Verlag von J. Cramer, 1967), reprint.

in a hot pan and rubbed to produce a powder which is applied to wounds.[35,36]

Uncaria tomentosa is commonly known to the Asháninka Indians as "samento." One ethnobotanist lists the plant as being used by the Asháninka to treat asthma, adding that the sap is mixed with water and drunk.[26] This species of cat's claw is also listed as one of the world's edible plants.[32] In Peru, *Uncaria tomentosa* is widely used among the Indians as an anti-inflammatory, contraceptive, and cytostatic (tumor-inhibiting) medicine, and it has many of the same common names as *U. guianensis*.[33] Common names that may be specific for *U. tomentosa* in Peru include "chacruk" (Jivaro Indian), "jipotatsa," and "garabato amarillo."[30]

In Amazonian Peru, the bark of *U. guianensis* is boiled to make a tea used to treat diabetes,[37] urinary tract cancer in women, cirrhosis, gastritis, and rheumatism.[33] In Huancabamba in northwestern Peru, shamans use *U. tomentosa* in much the same way; the bark is boiled and the tea is taken to treat gastric ulcers, rheumatism, inflammations, and tumors, and is also used as a contraceptive.[31]

The Cashibo Indians of eastern Peru have used cat's claw since ancient times. At night, when the moon is full, elders of the tribe pass their tradition of medicine on to the young. The following day, apprentices are taken into the forest and shown the plants they learned about the night before. Knowledge of cat's claw among the Cashibo has been passed on the same way for centuries. The bark tea is used to treat fevers and "loose stomach." The Cashibo believe the tea "normalizes the body." They also use the leaves of cat's claw as a cure for abscesses. Taking pieces of the leaves to form a small hand-rolled poultice, they place the leaf-ball into the abscess. They believe that by using the leaf "the body is clean."[13]

Medical anthropologists have found numerous applications of cat's claw in Peru. In addition to those uses noted above, they include hemorrhages, "impurities of the skin," blood purification, and irregularity of the menstrual cycle. And, like the bark, the leaves are believed to hold contraceptive properties.[13]

Traditional Uses of Cat's Claw

Uncaria guianensis	*Uncaria tomentosa*
Cancer (female urinary tract)[33]	Abscesses (leaf poultice)[13]
Cirrhosis[33]	Arthritis[43]
Contraception[31]	Asthma (sap with water)[26]
Diabetes[37]	"Blood purification"[13]
Dysentery (leaf extract)[35,36]	"Bone pains"[43]
Gastric ulcers[31]	Cancer[43]
Gastritis[31]	Chemotherapy side-effects[43]
Gonorrhea[33]	Contraception[3,13]
Inflammation[31]	Disease prevention[43]
Intestinal affections (infants)[35,36] (leaf extract)	Fevers[13]
Rheumatism[31]	Gastric ulcers[43]
Tumors[31]	Hemorrhages[13]
Wounds (leaf poultice)[35,36]	Inflammations[43]
	Kidney cleanser[43]
	Menstrual irregularity[13]
	"Normalizes the body"[13]
	Recovery from childbirth[43]
	Rheumatism[43]
	Skin "impurities"[13]
	Stomach ("loose")[13]
	Urinary tract inflammation[12]
	"Weakness"[43]
	Wounds[43]

Uncaria guianensis also grows in Bolivia, Brazil, Guyana, Paraguay, Trinidad, and Venezuela.[38] This species is described as a large climbing shrub that has "stout recurving spines," oval or elliptic leaves, "dry and nut-like" fruits (seeds), and small, dense white flowers that form a ball-shape at the end of long stalks.[39] But in Peru, red-orange flowers are found on

U. guianensis,[30] which tells us that botanists have yet to fully characterize this species.

The tiny flowers of *Uncaria tomentosa* are yellowish-white. Like those of *U. guianensis*, they cluster in a ball-shaped form at the top of the vine.[38] The seeds provide another means of distinguishing *Uncaria guianensis* from *U. tomentosa*. In *U. tomentosa*, the seeds are minute: 2.5-3.5 millimeters long and less than 1 mm wide, whereas in *U. guianensis* the seeds are about 4-8 mm in length and about 1-2 mm wide.[30,40]

The range of *U. tomentosa* is extreme. Botanists have located the vine in Colombia, Ecuador, Guyana, Trinidad, Venezuela,[38] Suriname, and in Central America,[41] in Guatemala, Costa Rica, and Panama. One Panamanian name, *bejuco de agua*, means "from which we drink water." Because of the way it twists and winds itself around other plants to reach more sunlight, the vine "Rangayo" is regarded as a nuisance weed by banana growers on the Atlantic coast of Central America.[42]

Legend of the Asháninka

The Asháninka Indians of central Peru know many specific uses for the vine. At least one shaman uses the stalk bark of cat's claw as a kidney cleanser, for "bone pains," and to cure "deep wounds."[43] The bark tea is also employed to treat inflammations of the urinary tract.[13] Other tribes make similar use of *U. guianensis* in Amazonian Peru where this species is taken as a remedy for cancer of the female urinary tract.[33]

Asháninka women use cat's claw to "recover after childbirth." However, the bark is primarily administered to control inflammations, gastric ulcers, arthritis, rheumatism, and cancer. It is also recommended to relieve side-effects from chemotherapy, to assist the defenses of those on antibiotics, and to those who suffer from "weakness." In treating wounds, the tea is drunk and used externally as a wash applied twice daily. For serious diseases, the Asháninka take a liter of the tea a day for a mini-

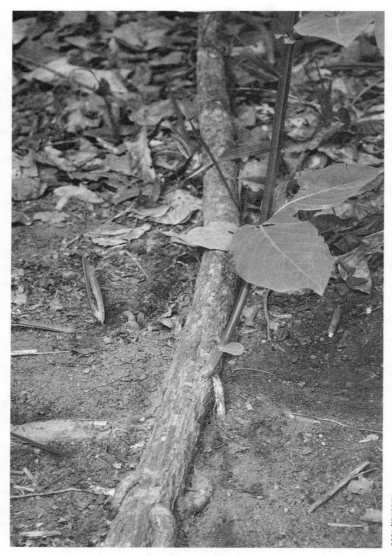

Uncaria tomentosa (Willd.) DC snaking along the ground at Brell's plantation. Note partly exposed secondary roots and new growth from the stalk.

K. Jones, 1995

mum of three months, "or until the symptoms or injuries have totally disappeared." To prevent diseases they recommend drinking a cup as often as once a week, or even once every 15 days.[43]

The indigenous peoples of Peru, including tribes of the Aguaruna, Asháninka, Cashibo, Conibo, and Shipibo, have been using *Uncaria tomentosa* for at least 2,000 years.[13] Today, cat's claw is mostly associated with the Asháninka ('aSHAninka'), an indigenous people of the Peruvian central rainforest who presently number about 50,000.[44] They are also the most recognized commercial source of cat's claw, an achievement attributable to their superior organization in harvesting and processing the vine and, also, to direct access to cat's claw in their homelands of central Peru.[13]

The Asháninka were the only tribe in Peru not conquered by the Incas. Through most of the last three centuries they remained hostile and resistant to exploitation. Their pride, willingness to fight, and location on the eastern side of the Andes across miles of jungle and rivers, all worked to keep missionaries, settlers, and soldiers away. Much to their credit, this proud tribe refused to tolerate mistreatment by either the land barons or in the form of religious laws imposed on them. As late as 1870, there were still numerous "war-like" Asháninka who hated the white people and were even feared by other tribes.[25] Today, even with the menace and degradation of the narco-terrorists, the Asháninka reputation for valor and self-possession remains largely intact.[45]

The Asháninka also use the water available in the center of the vine to treat diseases and this liquid is taken as a refreshing drink that "gives life."[43] The idea of the vine as a life-giving plant can be traced to an Asháninka legend about "samento" which tells how it came to be used by the tribe in the first place. It was recently retold by Chief Raul Vega of the Valle Esmeralda Asháninka community in the Ene River Valley[46] which is located near the center of Peru:

"The moon is Kashiri, supreme god of the Asháninka. The legend tells that one night in which Kashiri lit up the heavens, an Asháninka hunter went along a narrow path looking for prey to sustain his family. Already exhausted after many hours of fruitless searching, thirst and desperation diminished the strength of the solitary wayfarer.

Suddenly, a whispering in the woods called his attention and great was his surprise upon seeing an enormous otorongo [jaguar] tearing with his claws the bark from a thick vine.

Timidly but with curiosity, the man observed how the otorongo drank the water that issued from the heart of the vine. Then he saw how the otorongo, with ferocity and great agility, threw himself upon a deer that was casually passing by.

Awakened by this scene, the hunter silently drew near the vine and drank from the powerful water.

Minutes later, the hunter felt himself newly full of vigor, and decided to take a piece of bark from this vine that, curiously, had spines similar to that of the otorongo. Already it had dawned, and an enormous sachavaca [tapir] crossed his path. With an arrow directly to the heart, the hunter took his sachavaca's life.

Afterwards the Asháninka valued and used this vine which they called samento or uña de gato, a plant with curative, magical, and revitalizing powers.

It is because of it [samento] that the Asháninka fear the otorongo [jaguar], but never hunt it, else the god, Tasorentsi, be bothered and leave them to die of hunger and sickness."[47]

For serious diseases, the Asháninka mix the vine with other botanical medicines, such as "sangre de drago" and the bark of a tree called "chuchuhuasi" (*Maytenus* species). I also learned that it is traditionally the women of the tribe who know how to administer the vine and know which plants to combine it with in treating serious diseases.[43] That wasn't surprising, but it became something else to inquire about in Peru, to say nothing of these other plants. The fact that sangre de drago or "dragon's blood" had come to my attention twice now in relation to cat's claw clearly suggested a need to revisit the library for more research before I could reasonably begin my trip. (See appendix: Plants Combined with Cat's Claw.)

The Asháninka believe in using the bark fresh, "because its curative properties are reduced over time." They prepare the shredded bark of cat's claw as a tea by boiling about an ounce in a quart or so of water. The bark is left to boil for at least 15 minutes and may be taken warm, hot, or cold throughout the day. It can also be sweetened with sugar or honey. The more traditional method, in which the Asháninka boil pieces of the bark scraped from the stalk in a little water for a minimum of one hour, is much simpler. After it is prepared, the tea is typically taken cold throughout the day. The only precaution they make involves drinking too much — roughly three times the recommended amount — which can cause a loose stool. That problem is easily eliminated by drinking plenty of water instead of the tea over a period of two days.[43]

One authority on Peruvian medicinal plants, Dr. Fernando Cabieses, explains that in extremely large amounts *U. tomentosa* is used by Asháninka women as a contraceptive. He says they boil 11-13 pounds of the root in water until the liquid reduces to a little more than a cup. The decoction is then taken for three months during the period of menstruation. Cabieses adds that according to an Asháninka woman whose father was a shaman, by correctly using this drink, women "do not become pregnant for three to four years."[3]

In the course of preparing for Peru, I learned that a contraceptive effect was something Austrian scientists had begun to test cat's claw for in 1982. What they tested was a water extract of the pulverized root of *U. tomentosa*. While they established that the root was non-toxic, they also found that after mice drank a water extract at a rate of 6.25 milligrams per kilogram of their body weight, when females were caged with males, zero offspring were produced.[19] They offered no explanation as to why and didn't pursue the matter further, except to establish that alkaloid compounds in the root were not involved.[17] That was hardly proof the vine worked as a contraceptive, but it did raise the question of what prompted the Asháninka to use the root as a contraceptive in the first place. Perhaps they noticed the vine had stopped other kinds of growths.

Following a mandate from the President of Peru in 1995 to increase family planning, the National College of Chemistry suggested that use of cat's claw as a contraceptive by the Indians of Peru should be thoroughly investigated. If it works, they want to see the use patented, along with the compounds responsible.[84] In such a Catholic country as Peru, even the idea of contraception is controversial. And yet, many would argue that if only one could be found, a safe and effective herbal contraceptive is exactly what our over-populated world needs.

———————

The contraceptive aspect of cat's claw reminded me of my conversations with Whitworth. He explained that Brell had some theory about herbs used as contraceptives and their potential to combat cancer. As Whitworth put it, Brell suspected that if a plant could prevent the development of a fetus, then it might also prevent the development of other "growths."[5] I pointed out that as strange as that may seem, this theory is well-known to oncologists, some of whom even go so far as to insist that the growth of a baby starts out as what could really be called a "fetaloma." These scientists have long-suspected that one day we would find contraceptive agents that would also prevent the formation of tumors.

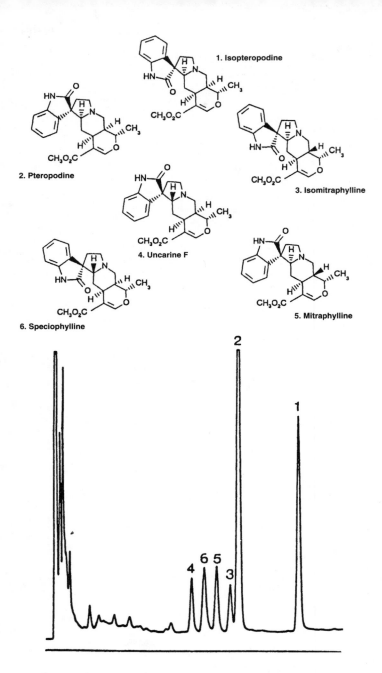

Chromatogram of oxindole alkaloids in a crude alcoholic extract of the root (*Uncaria tomentosa*). Adapted from Stuppner.[97]

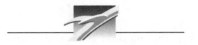

II.
Extracts and Actions

Long before I would venture to Peru, I had first to study what was published about the activity of the vine. So far, I had learned that cat's claw had a contraceptive activity. Its effects on the immune system were also something to investigate. Now I set out to learn which, among the numerous traditional uses of the vine by the Indians of South America, were known to have some basis from tests. I had every reason to be optimistic. For cancer alone, 70% of the plants found to hold antitumor activity were found in tropical forests.[85] Over 20 years of studies on cat's claw by Klaus Keplinger[7,19] was another good indication that I would be learning the vine held some definite activities against disease — activities presaged by the indigenous healers of Peru.

Twenty years is also the time it usually takes for a plant-derived medicinal product to go from the rainforest to the marketplace, and there have been some outstanding examples. For instance, the arrow poison curare was at one time only used in the jungles where Indian hunters delivered the extract at the point of an arrow to stun fish and game. Derived from the resin of a vine (*Chondrodendron tomentosum* Wedd.), curare is a very effective muscle relaxant. Pharmacologists found it held some valuable activities and now an alkaloid (tubocurarine) derived from the arrow poison saves lives in the treatment of spasms in spastic paralysis and those caused by tetanus. Little more than 10 years ago, surgeons found the alkaloid, and later derivatives made from it, invaluable in operations requiring the relaxation of muscles. Today, the alkaloid from the arrow poison is indispensable to surgeons all over the world.[86,87]

Cooling Inflammation

Knowing that most of the primary traditional uses of cat's claw involved inflammatory processes, this became the first topic I chose to explore.

Inflammation had been the topic of special focus in several studies of the vine and while perusing the library and data bases, I found that Italian and Peruvian scientists had teamed up to study this action in 1989. Using the bark of *U. tomentosa,* they found a very definite, although moderate, anti-inflammatory action in rats. They also examined a likely source of this action in sterols from the bark. Sterols are compounds chemically related to steroids. Most of the sterols were made up of *Beta*-sitosterol (60 %), a known natural anti-inflammatory compound found in small amounts in many plants. However, by themselves, the amount of sterols in the bark couldn't account for the amount of anti-inflammatory action that cat's claw had produced.[88]

Similar research had been conducted in Peru at the same time. Because cat's claw is used by the Indians to treat gastric ulcers, experiments with rats were performed to see whether the root bark might prevent the formation of ulcers. Rats given a water extract of the root bark (*U. tomentosa*) by the oral route were then subjected to stress factors. The extract was essentially the "tea" made according to traditional practice. Twenty grams of pulverized root bark was heated in a liter of water for 45 minutes at 185°F and allowed to cool in a refrigerator for 30 days before the tests began. Marco A. Costa Fazzi, of the Faculty of Medicine at the University of Cayetano Heredia in Lima, found three milliliters of the extract sufficient to cause a significant reduction in both the size and number of larger ulcers in rats. Complete prevention was too much to hope for and gastric bleeding was not reduced.[89] Even so, the results do suggest that the traditional use of cat's claw as a treatment rather than a preventive measure for gastric ulcers, may have merit.

In Italy at the University of Naples, much effort has been made to isolate the most active anti-inflammatory part of cat's claw. Rita Aquino and colleagues, having recognized the widespread use of the vine in Peru to treat arthritis and gastritis, set out to examine glycosides. This was a group of compounds that had previously been neglected in studies of cat's claw.[90] Glycosides are composed mainly of glucose, contain at least one other type of organic compound, and occur widely throughout the plant kingdom.

Dr. Aquino found the glycosides in cat's claw to be a rare type known as quinovic acid glycosides, and that they were present in both the root bark of *U. tomentosa* as well as the bark of *U. guianensis*.[37,90,91]

It was a compound with a structure never before seen in nature.

Breaking down the root bark extract of cat's claw (*U. tomentosa*), they isolated the active parts for further study. They found the first fraction or part of the extract held eight types of the glycosides and was the most active against inflammation. When given orally to rats, the glycoside-rich fraction inhibited the inflammation caused by swelling in the rats' paws by 46.8% — significantly more activity than that of any of the other fractions.[91]

Aquino discovered the most potent anti-inflammatory glycoside in the root bark of *U. tomentosa* and gave it the provisional name of quinovic acid glycoside number seven. It was a compound with a structure never before seen in nature. While the discovery of quinovic acid glycoside number seven was a great achievement, Aquino and colleagues were careful to point out that this single chemical was not responsible for *all* the anti-inflammatory action. Indeed, they had demonstrated the fact by using other compounds found in the root bark, some known to have potent anti-inflammatory activity, such as ursolic acid and oleanolic acid,[92,93] and some other glycosides of cat's claw. Yet glycoside number seven was even more potent.[91]

Months later, I learned that in Peru the inner stalk bark of *Uncaria guianensis* had been run through a series of similar tests. The water extract showed protective activity against the formation of gastric ulcers in rats. The alcoholic (methanol) extract wasn't as strong, but it did show more anti-inflammatory activity.[94]

From the perspective of native uses, what I found most interesting in Aquino's studies was the fact that a simple water extract of the root bark, given orally, was one of the most active yet least concentrated preparations they tested. Inflammation was inhibited by 41.2%, which wasn't much different from the rate of the powerful glycoside-rich fraction. More importantly, the dosage was far smaller and for a person weighing 70 kilograms, it would amount to a little less than six grams of root bark extract. Naturally, a concentrated extract (nine parts root bark to produce one part extract) was even more potent. Taken orally, that extract produced a 69.2% inhibition of inflammation and at a smaller dosage (50 mg/kg).[91]

But, after reviewing research conducted in Germany, it was obvious that another group of compounds in the root, besides quinovic acid glycosides, held potent anti-inflammatory activity.[19,95] Now I could see why the less concentrated whole bark extracts in Aquino's tests[91] were even more potent than the isolated glycosides. Clearly, the alkaloids were involved. (See table: Anti-inflammatory Activity.)

Anti-inflammatory Activity of Cat's Claw
(*Uncaria tomentosa*) Oral Dosages

Root bark[91]	Dosage	% Inhibition
Water extract	84.0 mg/kg	41.2
Glycoside fraction	4.2 mg/kg	46.8
Glycoside #7	20.0 mg/kg	33
Triterpene fraction	2.3 mg/kg	37.4
Root[19]		
Water extract	2 mg/kg	16
	3 mg/kg	33
	10 mg/kg	38
	100 mg/kg	42
Total alkaloids[95]		
(Prior to inflammation)	30 ml	39 (after 2.5 hr.)
		27.5 (after 5 hr.)
Total alkaloids		
(Anti-arthritic test)	10 ml/day X 5	17.1

Adapted from Aquino,[91] Keplinger,[19] and Kreutzkamp.[95]

Usually bitter-tasting compounds, alkaloids are noted for their often powerful effects and many have been used as drugs. In fact, about half the drugs used today derive from alkaloids.[87] Caffeine is an alkaloid from plants which belong to the same family as cat's claw (Rubiaceae). Other well-known alkaloids derived from plants include the pain-killers cocaine from *Coca* species and codeine from poppy plants (*Papaver* species), the stimulant and nasal decongestant ephedrine from species of *Epheðra*, the antimalarial quinine from the bark of *Cinchona* trees, the milk secretion stimulant chlorostigmine from

Chlorostigma species, and the anticancer drugs vinblastine for Hodgkin's disease and vincristine for childhood leukemia, both derived from the Madagascar periwinkle (*Catharanthus roseus*).[96] The kind of alkaloids that were found immunologically active in cat's claw are known as oxindole alkaloids. Six main ones are found in the root.[95,97]

Once I had entered the subject of cat's claw's alkaloids, I was confronted with an area of activity that I had studied before: plants that stimulate the immune system.[98] Here, at the very least, I hoped to find some reasonable explanation for why people believed the vine to be useful in treating cancer.

Actions on the Immune System

At the University of Munich in 1985, professor Hildebert Wagner established that in cell cultures and in animals, five of the main oxindole alkaloids of the root significantly enhanced the immune system. The alkaloids had increased the activity of immunological cells to destroy foreign cells by an action known as *phagocytosis* — a kind of cell-devouring activity by which debris and pathogens are removed from the system to protect and repair the body. In cell cultures, Wagner had shown these alkaloids were active in relatively small amounts (micrograms), whereas larger amounts were ineffective.[99]

In people, it would take only milligrams or even micrograms of these alkaloids to produce results. Nevertheless, the presence of one alkaloid in particular was important to achieve the optimum results. This was isopteropodine. This alkaloid alone had shown more activity than the total raw mixture of alkaloids of the root combined.[99,100]

In Europe, isopteropodine has been the standard for judging quality and potency of cat's claw for many years. However, pteropodine is also important because a portion of this alkaloid becomes isopteropodine under the influence of heat.[101] Since these alkaloids are critical for potency, I looked into this matter further.

Immunomodulating Alkaloids of
Uncaria tomentosa
(Percent increase in phagocytosis)

Micrograms/ml cells	10.0	01.0	0.10
Oxindole Alkaloid			
Speciophylline	18.5	26.0	35.3
Isorynchophylline	25.2	27.3	16.1
Isomitraphylline	27.0	27.0	19.4
Pteropodine	21.7	26.1	23.0
Isopteropodine	48.7	55.9	38.2
Total alkaloids	21.0	15.7	10.3
Water extract of root	21.8	24.1	05.7

Adapted from Wagner[99] and Keplinger.[100]

Total amounts of oxindole alkaloids vary in the root throughout the year.[95] Amounts found in root products sold in Europe have varied from half a milligram to five milligrams per gram.[102] Like the other alkaloids, isopteropodine occurs in the root, stalk bark, and leaves of *Uncaria tomentosa* in varying amounts throughout the year.[95,101,103] Generally, lesser amounts occur in the stalk bark and leaves. In *U. guianensis*, the amount of alkaloids that occur throughout the year appears to be less than in *U. tomentosa*.[95] In the bark and leaves of *U. guianensis*, sometimes alkaloids don't show up at all.[95,104]

The average rate that the stalk bark of *U. tomentosa* stimulates the immune system is "between 10% and 20%." The average rate of immune stimulation produced by the roots is 30% to

40%. Put another way, this means that the root increases immune cell activity 1.5 to as much as four times that of the stalk bark. The difference appears to depend on the concentration of isopteropodine in the final product, whether tea, extract, or extract powder.[104] (See appendix: A Look at the Leaves).

Improving on Tradition

The discovery of immunostimulating activity from the oxindole alkaloids of cat's claw soon led to product refinements. For example, it was determined that "effectiveness" of cat's claw products depended on the quantity of oxindole alkaloids and "the alkaloid pattern."[100] Austrian researchers found the presence of certain oxindole alkaloid types or structures important for optimum activity. This resulted in various proprietary preparations of the root, such as a spray, ointment, cream, and extracts with a standardized or consistent alkaloid content composed mostly of pentacyclic rather than tetracyclic alkaloids (rynchophylline and isorynchophylline).[7] The pentacyclic alkaloids in cat's claw are isopteropodine, pteropodine, speciophylline, mitraphylline, isomitraphylline, and uncarine F.

Standardized root extracts used by European clinicians contain 1.3 to 1.75% oxindole alkaloids. The pentacyclic alkaloids comprise about 97% of the total oxindole alkaloid content. The usual dose of the extract powder is 20 milligrams and in some cases 60 mg per day. The liquid extract contains 81 milligrams of oxindole alkaloids per liter and adults take 20 drops three times daily.[7]

Another refinement in the development of root extract products was to remove most of the phenolic tannins (largely the ones that tan or stain), while leaving in the clear catechin tannins. These tannins form a complex with the alkaloids and enhance their activity.[100] Products embodying refinements such as these are sold in Europe as "phytopharmaceuticals."

The research of cat's claw in Austria changed the herb from

an obscure folk medicine of uncertain worth to one of more defined potential in benefiting the immune system. For example, scientists found that the immune systems of both healthy and sick patients taking a standardized root product (97% pentacyclic alkaloids) showed increased numbers of active cells. Clinicians observed the effect in monocytes and granulocytes which take on the activity of macrophages when sufficiently stimulated.[19] Macrophages are the large cell-devouring or scavenging cells mentioned earlier. They are also one of the major defensive cells of the immune system. In battling against foreign organisms, macrophages take up the very front lines of attack. Monocytes become involved in immune responses to tissue damage. They travel through the blood stream to emergency sites where they envelope and help destroy intruding foreign cells.[114]

In normal people who consumed the root tea, the number of active monocytes increased from 33% to 50% in one week.

Another potential benefit became apparent upon closer examination. The root had activated monocytes, which in turn come to the aid of a group of white blood cells known as lymphocytes, better enabling them to increase in number and attack foreign cells when provoked.[19]

In normal people who consumed the root tea, the number of active monocytes increased from 33% to 50% in one week. As one might expect, there were many variables involved, such as the alkaloid content, starting numbers of immune cells, and the age of the individuals. For instance, in a man of 70, the initial monocyte count was 54% active cells. Seven days later the count reached 78%. In a woman of 42, the count went from 63.6% to 100%. Clinicians in Europe also observed that when subjected to a standardized root extract, red blood cells were dramatically less susceptible to breakdown. And in unhealthy cells exposed to the water extract, the number of malformations was greatly reduced.[19,115]

But what about cancer? Didn't any results show antitumor activity? I learned that in Brazil, in the 1970s, there was some interest in the alkaloid pteropodine. The Institute of Antibiotics at the Federal University of Pernambuco in Recife tested the alkaloid for antitumor activity in cancer cells and in animals with tumors; however, no action was found.[116]

From a closer reading of the literature, I learned that in high amounts the total alkaloids did produce some *direct* antitumor activity in isolated cancer cells (P388 lymphocytic leukemia and KB cells).[100] Recent tests using isolated cancer cells produced inhibition of various leukemia and brain tumor cells (neuroblastomas) utilizing much smaller amounts of the total or individual alkaloids.[7] But for *immunomodulation*, which is key to cat's claw's role as an adjunct to cancer treatments, only low doses of the alkaloids are effective.[100]

Physician's Accounts

In most of the recorded uses of cat's claw against cancer, patients have also had chemotherapy, radiation, surgery, or have taken some other herbal medications in addition. For serious diseases, the Asháninka use cat's claw in combination with chuchuhuasi and sangre de drago.[45] Brell had a formula of herbs with cat's claw,[5] and Maxwell's acquaintance used cat's claw as the main ingredient of a regimen of herbs, such as chanca piedra and sangre de drago[28] (see appendix). By the time I had combed the science behind the folklore of the vine, I found others in remission from cancer who had also used cat's claw, although usually in combination with other herbs or conventional treatments.

After years of experience with cancer patients, Austrian researchers have determined that cat's claw functions in a supportive role. Simply put, they explain that the alkaloids increase the ability of the immune system to react. Clinicians observed that when standardized root products were used, chemotherapy and radiation therapy were tolerated far better by their cancer patients. Studies in mice with cancer showed that in those given the extract the action of anticancer drugs was "intensified."[115]

In people with cancer, recovery appeared to be faster and some patients taking the root tea appeared better able to tolerate further conventional treatments needed to make a full recovery. This was evident in blood tests where the cell numbers in cancer patients on cat's claw didn't drop as far as those without the root.[115] In a patient with melanoma, for example, this benefit could be seen in immunoglobulins (cells that make antibodies) and bacteria-fighting leucocytes. The same held true for other cancer patients, including some afflicted with leukemia, Hodgkin's disease, osteosarcoma, carcinoma, and breast cancer.[19] Naturally, these observations will require further clinical studies before the preparations used can be judged effective.

Since the mid-1980s, physicians in Europe who have applied an alkaloid-rich cat's claw root tea in their practice have noted various kinds of benefits. Their collective observations offer incentive for clinical trials where changes due to the root can be more closely monitored and compared to controls to gauge efficacy.

By 1995, preliminary tests had been made with patients in Austria. For example, two patients who had gastritis received a water extract of the root for over three weeks. After only three days of treatment, they no longer complained of symptoms and upon further examination objective readings had normalized. The same therapy appeared equally successful in a patient with a duodenal ulcer and in two patients who suffered from rheumatism; benefits appeared after only a short period of treatment.[19]

From years of experience with the root tea, Austrian physicians have observed that, on average, stomach ulcers and gastric problems generally seem to show improvements following eight days. But for lasting results they have found it necessary for patients to take the tea for at least three months. They add that sometimes, after 12 weeks, patients on the extract experience what seems to be a worsening of symptoms. This may last for three weeks or more, but following this experience patients improve.[115] In Europe, some people also take the standardized extract for a period of two to three months during the autumn as a general preventive immunostimulant.[117]

In Europe, some people also take the standardized extract for a period of two to three months during the autumn as a general preventive immunostimulant.

In cases of uveitis, a painful infection of the eye, a minimum of one year's treatment was required before lasting relief from pain. Austrian physicians noted that some patients with multiple sclerosis also seemed to show improvement, and that after a year's treatment some serious cases of allergic asthma had also responded. They responded so well that the root seemed to commonly relieve symptoms for three years and more.[115]

The press would be expected to report details that clinicians in Europe could not. When someone sent me a clipping from a European magazine, I wasn't disappointed. I read that a 10-year-old boy in Innsbruck had begun to carry his head at an angle, one eye was squinting, and that he had no control over his motions. A clinic at the University of Innsbruck found the boy was suffering from a brain tumor. Because it was located in the brain stem, the tumor was inoperable. He received radiation and chemotherapy for eight months with no sign of improvement. Treatment with cat's claw root tea was started in

October, 1984. In December there was no indication that the tumor had grown any further. By May the following year, his leg reflexes were back and his squinting eye could be corrected with surgery. By November, the tumor was beginning to diminish and had encapsulated itself. The boy returned to active sports, playing music, and showed normal growth.[118]

While a brain tumor can more easily be discounted as the result of a placebo response,[119] the same magazine carried the account of a doctor in Innsbruck who, since the age of 57, had suffered with a particularly difficult form of leukemia. Chemotherapy and other treatments had apparently been of no help and his liver was greatly enlarged. His physician, an immunologist at the University of Innsbruck, then decided to try the root tea. What ensued seemed nothing short of a "miracle." His liver shrank to near normal; his blood counts stabilized; and chemotherapy was stopped. The doctor hadn't felt so good in years.[118]

Clinical Research

Controlled clinical studies in Europe are ongoing with a variety of proprietary products made from the root of cat's claw (*U. tomentosa*) cultivars raised in Peru. These standardized products have been approved for use in Austria and Germany according to laws governing pharmaceuticals and they may only be prescribed by a physician. They are specifically permitted in cases where it is necessary to avert life-threatening situations or those posing a "severe damage to health," when a physician cannot expect to achieve a comparable result from registered pharmaceuticals.[7]

The clinical use of these products in Austria and Germany is designated for diseases mainly caused by a "malfunctioning of the immune system." Such applications may include rheumatoid arthritis, allergies, and a "supporting therapy in the management of neoplastic diseases and infections with herpes viruses and retroviruses." To date, the clinical studies of these products remain largely unpublished, unfinished, or requiring larger numbers of patients[7] before the results can be judged by the medical community at large. Even so, after over 10 years of research there are optimistic signs they will be found effective in the treatment of some of the world's most anguishing diseases.

An extract powder taken in capsules has been used by patients for over eight years in Europe without showing "any signs of a toxic effect." For example, the extract may be prescribed to cancer patients two weeks prior to undergoing chemotherapy or radiation treatments. Physicians have prescribed the extract for relapsing cancer patients at double and triple the usual dosage of 20-60 mg/day without fear for their patients' safety. However, there are some warnings. For example, in the case of children under three, there is, as yet, no clinical experience with the extract, so as a precaution and in compliance with the pharmaceutical laws of Austria and Germany, they are not allowed the product.[7] (See appendix: Safety Concerns.)

All patients on the root preparations experienced increased vitality and suffered less from radiation and chemotherapy side-effects.

An observatory trial in cancer patients was conducted over a 10-year period in which 56 patients participated. Those patients who had cancers in the early stages of development fared the best, with some remaining in remission after 10 years. The best results were seen in patients with testicular teratoma who had also received chemotherapy, and in patients with adenocarcinoma of the colon who had surgery in addition to using proprietary root products—a root tea (60 milliliters/day) or a powdered extract.[7]

The tea was made by heating 20 grams of pulverized root at 176°F for 45 minutes in a liter of cold water. An enamel vessel was advised and any losses to the liter from boiling were made up with added water. After allowing the tea to cool 10 minutes, it was poured through filter paper and stored in a tightly sealed container at 35.6-46.4°F. The root decoction produced was prescribed at the usual adult dose of 60 ml in 60 ml of hot water before breakfast.[7]

A more recent study in 60 patients suffering from various kinds of brain tumors was conducted at the Department of Neurosurgery at the Innsbruck Clinic, in Austria, from February 1990 to September 1991. All patients received chemotherapy, radiation, and surgery, in addition to root preparations after discharge from the clinic. The root preparations were not advised for use at the same time as chemotherapy, but only between treatments—two days prior and afterwards at every two to six days in alternation. The patients received a specially prepared liquid extract of the root in addition to a standardized extract powder (60 mg/day). One year later, in September 1992, the patients were examined to see how many had survived. Only 17 remained. All patients on the root preparations experienced increased vitality and suffered less from radiation and chemotherapy side-effects. The best results appeared in remissions in five out of six cases of ependymoblastoma (grades II and III), and in six out of eight cases of astrocytoma (grade II).[7] The survival rate for astrocytomas up to five years is about 10-20%. For blastomas, the five-year survival rate (disease-free) is 77% for lower risk patients and 39% for those at higher risk.[119]

Clinical or observational studies of standardized proprietary root extracts in Europe have also been made with patients suffering from leukemia, rheumatoid arthritis, allergic respiratory diseases (allergic asthma and hay fever), ulcers, gastritis, AIDS, and other viral diseases, such as *Herpes simplex* and

Herpes zoster (shingles). Using topical preparations of the root extract such as creams, ointments, and sprays in the treatment of *Herpes simplex* infections appeared very effective. In one study, pains were eliminated in 14 out of 17 patients by the third day and all patients by the seventh day. Relatively small amounts of the extract had previously shown a high degree of activity against genital *Herpes simplex* cells (94% inhibition from 3 micrograms of extract/ml of cells). And in mice, a topical solution (10%) of the extract caused a 40% reduction in *Herpes simplex* and accelerated the rate of healing from the infection. Therefore, positive results in patients are not surprising.[7]

When these studies are repeated in larger groups of patients and with additional controls, the information will be much more meaningful. I suspect that within a few years some of these diseases will undergo the clinical research needed and the results will be published for all the world to know.

An Anti-leukemic Component

In 1993, at the 41st Annual Congress on Medicinal Plant Research in Düsseldorf, Germany, the Department of Internal Medicine at the University of Innsbruck presented a brief report of their findings with cat's claw against leukemia. They reported they had taken six of the main alkaloids in cat's claw and tested them in cultures of leukemia cells. Dr. Hermann Stuppner explained that what they found was an ability of specific oxindole alkaloids to inhibit the proliferation of these cells.[120]

Stuppner found that all but one (mitraphylline) of the main oxindole alkaloids of cat's claw were active. The most active, by far, was uncarine F, another of the pentacyclic alkaloids. Unlike many of the anti-leukemic drugs, at the concentrations needed for this action, uncarine F didn't inhibit new immune cells from forming in stem cells. Normal stem cells, which are bone marrow cells that become cells of the immune system, were left unharmed. The very selective nature of uncarine F brought Stuppner to suggest that this alkaloid might, at least, be considered by those in search of new drugs to combat acute leukemia.[120]

One of the possible mechanisms of the antileukemic activity that Stuppner found could involve something known as DNA polymerase, an enzyme system that allows abnormal cells to proliferate. Researchers in Italy have found that extracts of cat's claw (*U. tomentosa*) inhibit this enzyme system—an action that in turn inhibits abnormal cells from growing.[121] Other independent Austrian researchers are currently studying various alkaloids and components of the root on different types of leukemic cells.[7]

Catechin Tannins

The most mysterious aspect of cat's claw lies in the fact that an immunologically inactive compound, a kind of tannin in the plant, still makes a significant contribution to immunological activity. In one of those synergistic effects where the sum seems to be greater than its individual parts, catechin tannins in the root contribute 10% of the immunoactivity. Yet, by themselves, they are inactive on the immune system.[100]

From a crude water extract of the root without these tannins, the rate of increased immune activity in rodents was 1.7. With the catechin tannins the rate increased to 2.3, but no one knows why.[100] They may serve as so-called carrier substances—delivering the alkaloids to the system in some manner that science has yet to fully understand. But, what science does know about these tannins could tell us something more about the actions of cat's claw.

Cat's claw is a rich source of tannins. One kind of catechin tannin found in the dried root bark of cat's claw is *cis*-epicatechin.[116] This type of catechin has shown potent antioxidant activity, even more potent than vitamin E. There is even some evidence suggesting that epicatechin may protect the small blood vessels of the brain from damage caused by free radical electrons.[122]

Tannins do a lot more than stain tea cups. Because tannins are found throughout the plant kingdom, their actions are fundamental to the use of herbal teas. For example, tannins modify the secretion of bile in the liver and can aid in the absorption of other active plant substances simply by inhibiting movement in the intestines.[123] Catechin tannins have long been known to protect vitamin C from oxidizing,[124,125] and there are indications that these tannins can form complexes with red blood cells which can then contribute to the responses of the immune system.[126]

Catechin tannins are well-known for their astringent or tissue-contracting action which gives medicinal plants abundant in these tannins common uses as wound-healing and antidiarrheal agents. In traditional medicine, rich sources of catechin tannins, especially woody plants, are used to treat nose-bleeds, ulcers, boils, burns, and hemorrhoids.[127]

As part of a large group of naturally occurring chemicals in plants called flavonoids, catechin tannins are of great interest to scientists studying the effects of diet on cancer. Research has shown that flavonoids can inhibit the formation of cancers by an antioxidant action that protects the body's cells from processes of cellular decay and damage caused by free radicals. Cellular oxidation is the process whereby cells are broken down by reactive types of oxygen composed of unpaired electrons known as free radicals. Many food scientists reason that by taking antioxidants our cells will have a better chance of staying healthy.[127-129]

Researchers in the Netherlands have found the main source of flavonoids in the diet of their country is tea.[128] One can expect that to be the case in many countries. Not only is a significant portion of the flavonoids in green and black tea made up of catechin tannins, but they have also been found to inhibit the formation of tumors.[129,130] Researchers are now examining the diet for total flavonoids and catechin tannin content. They want to see whether intake levels might affect the incidence of cancers. Investigators in Japan have already found the catechin tannins in green tea have an antimutagenic effect. This action alone could lower the incidence of cancer. By protecting normal cells from being mutated into abnormal ones as a result of dietary factors or environmental toxins, antimutagens could reduce the chance of cells becoming cancerous.[131]

The other important tip is to prepare herbal teas with finely ground material and allow the heat used in making the tea enough time to liberate the active constituents.

Studies show that to gain the most flavonoids from herbal teas, the material needs to be powdered before boiling. The time allowed for boiling is also important. Provided the teas are prepared at 212°F, 30 to 45 minutes produces a high level of flavonoids from herbs.[132]

Another advantage to this method of preparation is increased assimilation in the digestive tract. Patients using herbal teas, who showed clinical improvements, were found to have a much greater level of antioxidant activity in their gastric juices.[135] In their article titled "Why are Natural Plant Medicinal Products Effective in Some Patients and not in Others with the Same Disease?" researchers at the Niwa Institute for Immunology in Kochi-ken, Japan, concluded those patients who could more easily break down herbal products in their digestive system had the best clinical results. They also concluded that the antioxidant activity from the flavonoids released through heating medicinal plant materials appears to provide a greater advantage to patients.[133,134]

To date, little work has been devoted to the flavonoids in cat's claw. One of the earliest investigations found five procyanidins (A1, B1, B2, B3 and B4) in the root bark.[116] Procyanidins—a subclass of larger compounds known as proanthocyanidins—are water-soluble flavonoids well-known for their anti-inflammatory activity. In clinical research, procyanidins have shown a strengthening effect on collagen fibers in connective tissue and they appear to promote collagen formation. They protect and strengthen the veins and are prescribed in Europe to treat varicose veins and weaknesses of the eyes, whether from eye-stress, fatigue, or simply age. Procyanidin-rich topical preparations are used to protect the skin and hair from sun damage, which is largely caused by free radicals.[135]

Together, catechin tannins and procyanidins contribute an antioxidant and radioprotective activity[51,135] which would help to protect normal cells from the damaging effects of chemotherapy and radiation. Procyanidins, alone, have shown potent anti-inflammatory, antimutagenic, radioprotective, and antioxidant effects. Since the antioxidant activity of procyanidins is much more potent than that of vitamin E or of catechin tannins,[135] these components may be critical to traditional uses of cat's claw in Peruvian folk medicine. In a preliminary analysis, one independent laboratory found substantial amounts of procyanidins in cat's claw. A commercial stalk bark contained 12% procyanidins and an extract powder of this bark contained 48% procyanidins.[136]

Looking to early Austrian studies with the root, I couldn't help but notice that doctors there understood what worked best long before the digestive studies with herbal teas in Japan. They noted that patients with poor levels of stomach acids weren't able to take full advantage of the alkaloids.[115] Now the latest research on assimilation of herbs indicates that levels of pepsin and acid in the gastric juices are critical for assimilating the antioxidant compounds.[132,133] The other important tip is to prepare herbal teas with finely ground material and allow the heat used in making the tea enough time to liberate the active constituents.[133] For cat's claw, allow 45 minutes to an hour or more.[45,93]

Mutation Management

The theme of leaving normal cells normal was repeated in research with the root bark of cat's claw (*U. tomentosa*).[137,138] Three universities in Italy collaborated on a study of possible antimutagenic effects. Dr. Renato Rizzi of the University of Milan headed up the study. They wanted to see whether cat's claw could inhibit the mutation of normal cells,[121] an action that would, as a matter of course, help to prevent disease, particularly cancer.

After extensive testing, no mutagenic effects from the root bark could be found. However, the antimutagenic effect was significant. In one test, they used *Beta*-carotene for comparison. Well-known for its antimutagenic action, *Beta*-carotene is the yellow-orange coloring matter found in carrots, other vegetables, and some fruits, such as the mango. In equal amounts, a water extract of the root bark reduced by half the number of cells that would have mutated. For *Beta*-carotene the figure was 68%. When an extract of cat's claw made with an alcoholic solvent was tested, mutation was inhibited by 59%. Obviously, the alcohol had liberated more of the active components.[139]

Cat's claw could now be listed among the other natural substances of the world known as antimutagens.[139] Among them are vitamins, such as vitamins A, C, and E, and flavonoids, such as catechin tannins[129,130] and procyanidins.[136] But would that activity hold up in people? Ironically, a study to find out was made in people who were exposed to smoke daily—the very factor that, years ago, set Brell to pondering the cancer preventive effect of cat's claw in the diet.[4]

Before a larger clinical study is conducted, scientists perform smaller pilot studies to see whether the effects observed in the laboratory will even begin to hold up in people. Dr. Rizzi and colleagues used the same approach. Two healthy individuals, who would drink the root bark tea, were selected. Because smokers are known to produce mutated cells in their urine, one subject was a smoker and the other a non-smoker. Both were 35-year-old men and the smoker had used about 20 cigarettes a day for more than 15 years. They made sure these subjects had not been treated with X-rays or drugs for more than six months, they didn't have any viral diseases, and they hadn't been working with chemicals that could cause cancer.[139] Any of those factors could have produced mutated cells in the urine, which was what the researchers were about to test.

Following traditional methods for making the tea, they made a decoction by boiling dry root bark for three hours, at which time the amount of liquid was reduced to one-third. Both men drank about 6.5 grams of the tea a day for 15 days. Urine was collected before, during, and after the test. At the start, the non-smoker's urine had no mutagenic activity and that persisted during and after drinking the tea. The smoker had mutagenic activity in his urine before the test, but the activity diminished rapidly during the time he drank the tea and even for eight days later.[139]

The point of this study was not to find an excuse for smokers, but to learn whether cat's claw might hold antimutagenic activity for the benefit of everyone. The second point of the study was to begin to get some idea of the parts responsible for the antimutagenic action. Dr. Rizzi reasonably suspected components with antioxidant activity.[139]

Antioxidation

Antioxidants inhibit the oxidation or "burning up" of cells. Synthetic and natural antioxidants are added to foods as preservatives for the same reason: they function as scavengers of unpaired electrons called free radicals—cell-damaging electrons capable of mutating unprotected cells and of causing foods to deteriorate and spoil. There are numerous sources of free radicals. Chemotherapy agents and X-rays are two of the most powerful and it is partly because of the free radicals they produce that they are able to arrest the growth of cancer cells. The problem is, free radicals often escape and their damage to normal cells can lead to cancer later on. Much less powerful but damaging sources of free radicals are found in air pollution, smoke, pesticides, alcohol, vigorous and frequent exercise, too much sunlight, and too much dietary fat. These facts are well-known today. Because of this, millions of people now take antioxidant supplements such as *Beta*-carotene and vitamins A, C, and E on a regular basis.[140-143]

There are other instances of medicinal plants having an antimutagenic effect which is partly due to tannins.[144] In some cases, the degree of antioxidant and free radical scavenging activity of medicinal plant extracts is even greater than vitamins C or E, which are two of the best dietary antioxidants known.[122,145,146] Besides catechin tannins and procyanidins,[116] cat's claw contains oleanolic and ursolic acids (triterpenes),[89] both scavengers of free radicals.[147] What other components might be involved in the cell-protective effects of cat's claw await further research. Not only are there many kinds of antioxidants in plants,[148] but protective mechanisms could also result from immunological processes.

PERU

Iquitos

Lima

Machu Picchu

ANDES

ASHÁNINKA TERRITORY

Rio Pozuzo

Rio Pachitea

Rio Pichis

Rio Ucayali

Rio Urubamba

Pozuzo

Puerto Bermudez

Rio Nevati

Oxampampa

Rio Chanchamayo

Villa Rica

Pichanaki

Rio Perené

Rio Tambo

La Merced

San Ramón

Rio Tarma

Satipo

Rio Ene

Cutivireni

Rio Mantaro

N

0   30   60
        Miles

R. Rawling, 1995

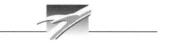

III.
Guide to Uña de Gato

After reviewing the information available on the activity and traditional uses of cat's claw, I had little hope of finding much more to add from a visit to Peru. However, there were still critical questions that I needed to answer. The ecology of the vine was high on my list. Rumors of cat's claw becoming endangered from over-harvesting in Peru were circulating in the marketplace, as were allegations of the root being illegal to export. In the end, I limited my list to unpublished studies, regulatory and ecological matters, and the one thing that held my curiosity the most, the pioneering work of Arturo Brell.

Through a series of fortuitous setbacks, I was able to contact the living descendants of Brell just weeks before my flight to Peru, even though Whitworth had lost all means of contact years ago. I was delighted to find that Brell's granddaughter, Guisella Tesoro Brell, was not only a serious biologist, but one actively engaged in propagation studies of the vine. We arranged to meet in the town of La Merced located in the Province of Chanchamayo, a thriving agricultural area in central Peru.

During the long flight from Los Angeles to Lima, I began to feel a definite kinship with Peruvians. I attribute this to growing up in Canada, which, like Peru, is a highly multicultural society. This feeling grew stronger when I met my guides the following day. I was amazed to learn that one of them was an old friend of Nicole Maxwell, the American ethnobotanist who wrote about cat's claw in her book, *Witch Doctor's Apprentice*

(Citadel Press, 1990). The guides were associates of my publisher and offered to take me across the Andes the very next day. For selfless reasons they choose to remain anonymous.

The morning after my arrival in Lima, we would travel due east for about 150 miles. Our biggest hurdle to reach my destination would be the journey over the Andes. The tour only seemed to begin when we stopped at a roadside cafe. At an elevation of about 10,000 feet, I began to feel the effects of the altitude. I was feeling only a little more resilient after two pots of coca-leaf tea. The thin mountain air still made me dizzy and, if not for the dramatic scenery, I could have fallen asleep at any moment.

We had been winding and climbing for hours when, through the red and purple hues of a towering mountain pass, we could finally see the snowy crowns of the high Andes. It was our reward and incentive to move on, but there was always a good excuse to stop. A few pigs, a rushing stream, or a patch of bright green grass beside an old brick hut, and my camera needed feeding again. My generous guides didn't mind a bit.

When we reached the point of 16,000 feet above sea level, the truck began to sputter and jerk as the carburetor gasped for oxygen. Outside, it was so cold that it seemed like winter in Canada. Now at the top of our climb, we had finally left the gray skies that cover most of the coast during the winter in August. The sky ahead of us was blue, and in my destination of the Chanchamayo Valley, I knew the season was summer.

Our descent was like slipping backwards in time. The fields of crops that Andean people had quilted into the hills of the dry highlands centuries ago were just as they had first built them. Llamas roamed, with brightly clothed caretakers nearby, and the old Spanish buildings in the towns seemed scarcely changed. When at last we reached the valley below, I felt my lungs expand from the increase in oxygen produced by the greater density of plants. It was a dramatic demonstration of just how diverse the climatic zones of Peru really are. Then came the buzzing of huge insects and I knew the jungles

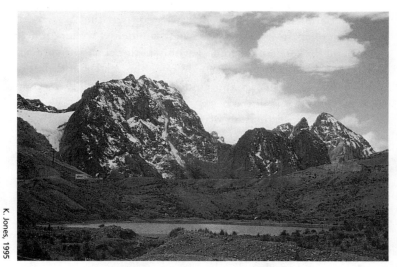

K. Jones, 1995

The Andes at the top of our climb from Lima.

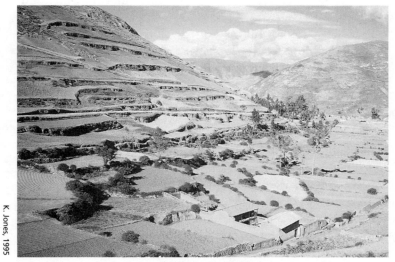

K. Jones, 1995

Ancient Andean fields along the descent to the Chanchamayo Valley.

couldn't be far away. Their noise was so loud that we could hear them over the sound of the truck. Suddenly, banana trees, palms, and flowers most people see only in florist shops were all around us. Our roller coaster ride over the Andes and down into the jungle wasn't in any guidebook that I had ever seen, yet it was surely one of the best.

Reaching my destination of La Merced, I found a room in one of the larger hotels. It was still early evening and I marveled at how far we had come in such a short time and over so much different terrain and climate. The air was hot and the odor of produce was everywhere. While we waited for the Brells at a nearby restaurant, passing soldiers cast a wary eye, while Shipibo Indians approached to sell their wares. Finally, the moment for which I had traveled to Peru was at hand. As Brell's granddaughter Guisella appeared with her husband and mother to greet us, I realized I was now directly linked to the dim past of cat's claw in Peru. The surprise that Guisella and her mother kept for my arrival was that they would allow me to access Brell's archives. They contained documents which few people had ever seen.

Exhausted from a full day of traveling, we decided to save our conversations for the days ahead. Arrangements were made to visit Brell's old plantation the following morning and we said goodnight.

Surveying the Vines

Daylight arrived with the incessant noise of bus drivers calling out their destinations. It was barely 5:00 AM and the sounds of the marketplace told me I may as well get out of bed. Across the street it was like a carnival. The stalls were brimming with fresh oranges, sacks of coffee, crates of mangos, avocados, pineapples, cacao, taro root, peanuts, sugar cane, and more kinds of potatoes than most people could imagine. The herb stalls were just as rich with cat's claw, chuchuhuasi, chanca piedra, and other diverse medicinal plants.

As the sun climbed over the palm-trimmed hills, the smell of coffee and fruit filled the morning air. Guisella arrived with her mother, Elfriede, and husband, Jim, while I was finishing breakfast and preparing my camera. Brell's great-granddaughter, Kim, was there, too. Elfriede had just learned the doctor I wanted to find—the one from Lima who had led Whitworth to Brell—was visiting the Province of Chanchamayo, too. When I contacted Guisella before arriving in Peru, she had not known who the doctor was or where I could find him. At the time, no one was sure the doctor was still alive, including Whitworth, who couldn't even recall his name. Guisella's mother put out the word among old friends; we wanted to see him before I had to leave for Lima. There was no guarantee we would meet, yet we were hopeful.

Our mutual quest could not have been more timely. Together, we were about to follow any leads we could to Arturo Brell's storied past with cat's claw. Now studying the very life of the vine that her grandfather had devoted himself to, for Guisella it was a history that had become considerably more than a curiosity. On the way to the plantation I caught glimpses of a river nearby where I could see Indians fishing and washing, just as their ancestors had done. Passing miles of plantations teeming with avocados, cacao, coffee, limes, and oranges, I tried to get a sense of what the immigrants to Chanchamayo must have felt when they arrived from Europe nearly a century ago. The beauty was restful. However, in earlier times the area was far more lush, and for Brell and the other earlier settlers, the fertile, undisturbed valley must have been a garden of peace and opportunity. Today, the population has reached 113,000 and there seems to be no end to the crops that will grow. Recently, macadamia nuts and silk worms were introduced.

As the sun rose higher, it was getting awfully hot in a hurry. The drive was far longer than I anticipated, but just when it seemed we would never find the place, the lead vehicle came to a stop. We walked the rest of the way down a broad path.

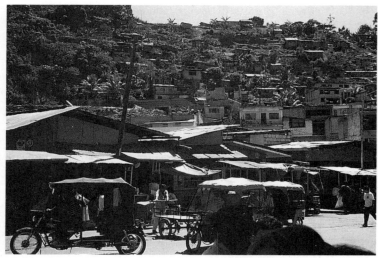

K. Jones, 1995

Morning rush-hour in downtown La Merced.

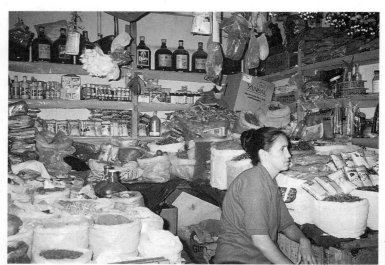

K. Jones, 1995

A herb stall in La Merced.

Upon entering the grounds, Guisella casually mentioned that one entrance of the neglected old house I saw before me was once the Whitworth-Brell Research Institute. Somewhere inside Guisella found the old sign that hung over the Institute entrance. I could hardly wait to tell Whitworth. Not only had I kept my promise of finding the old clinic, I could confidently report that despite the heliport having been reclaimed by the jungle, the canoe port and the donkey port were like new.[149]

The land was filled with overgrown fruit trees. Brell had planted nearly all of them, decades ago. There were towering avocados, huge mangoes, some old coffee bushes, and oranges as far as the eye could see. A gentle breeze from the river nearby helped me to stay comfortable long enough to fumble for my film. Guisella explained that Brell's old plantation had once been the site of an Indian village. Shards of Indian pottery protruded from the soil of a steep bank overlooking the river. Hoping that one day the site might be attended by an archeologist, we left the relic just as we found it.

Elfriede was a little girl when Whitworth and his team arrived at the plantation on their expedition in the 1960s. She also remembered Keplinger. He was the Austrian journalist who had spent a whole year traveling extensively in the area in 1974. She gave me a copy of an article from a German newspaper from 1965, where I read that Brell had been experimenting with cat's claw even earlier.[9,149]

During his first visit to Bavaria in 40 years, Brell was interviewed by a local newspaper about his life in Peru. He was described as an open-minded individual with many interests and one who solved the practical and human problems of frontier life by relying on his own common sense. Like all German immigrant landowners in Peru during the Second World War, he was forced to give up his property and "disappear" into the jungles. Asháninka Indians he befriended came to his aid until the war ended. For Brell, who would now have the chance to observe the ways of the Asháninka more closely, this was a time of different opportunities.[9] His childhood dream of studying the ancient culture of Peru[4] was now at hand.

He observed that the women who took this bark for years had "healthy and strong children, whom they naturally breast-fed."

Brell noticed that the Asháninka women customarily used the bark of a particular vine as a kind of herbal birth control. The name they gave this vine sounded like "zavenna rozza." The bark was taken once a month in the form of a decoction (boiled preparation). Brell reported it seemed to be free of side-effects and, regardless of long-term use, there was no sterilization. He observed that the women who took this bark for years had "healthy and strong children, whom they naturally breast-fed." He also noted the men made a habit of drinking the same bark tea, simply because their instincts led them to believe it would do them "good."[9]

Brell also took special notice of their constant exposure to wood-smoke. All day long they fanned the smoke of their fires to ward off insects. And yet, despite their life-long chronic exposure to tars and ash, to his knowledge they never had cancer. When Brell reasoned the bark tea might be affording them some kind of protection,[9] his research of the vine we know today as cat's claw really began. Eventually, Brell developed several formulas based on cat's claw as the main ingredient. There was a formula for serious diseases such as cancer, one for retarding the aging process, and another for preventing disease.[149] In keeping with his wishes and long before they ever become released to the public, these formulas deserve intense scientific evaluation. To do otherwise would neither credit Brell for his work, nor allow him the respect he deserved.

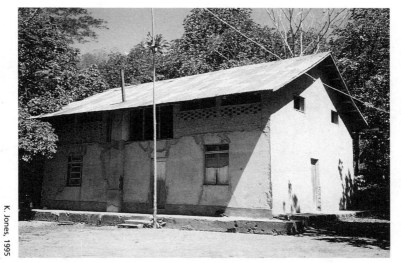

K. Jones, 1995

The house of Arturo Brell and the Whitworth-Brell Research Institute, Chanchamayo, Peru.

The old plantation was Elfriede's childhood home and it was full of memories for Guisella, too. The house was still in good shape and I could tell it wouldn't take much to fix up. Guisella agreed and told me that it was a dream of hers to restore the plantation and to establish some kind of botanical research center, perhaps one where visitors such as myself could stay and study medicinal plants.[150]

She walked me over to see the vines that her grandfather had planted some 40 years earlier. Stunning to behold, one measured over 90 feet in length. There was *Uncaria tomentosa* and *Uncaria guianensis*. Guisella couldn't believe my luck. In the forest canopy above, I could see the yellowish flowers of the *tomentosa* in full bloom.

The strength of these woody vines is remarkable. I found Elfriede sitting on the bow of one as if it were a swing. When I dared to sit next to her, she told me the vine would hold. She gave a push with her feet and we were swinging on the vine

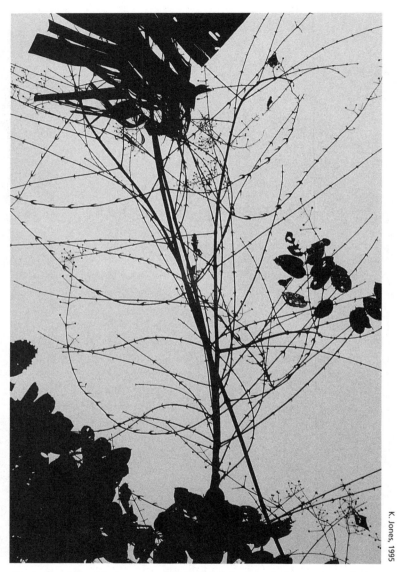

K. Jones, 1995

The ends of *Uncaria tomentosa* (Willd.) DC clawing their way through the forest canopy in Chanchamayo, Peru.

with our full weight. Guisella explained that cat's claw can take 10 years to grow to a size large enough to be harvested for bark, and that the vine I was swinging on (*Uncaria tomentosa*) was at least 30 years old.[150]

At the point where I sat with Elfriede, the vine had climbed down from a supporting mango tree before climbing up another tree across a distance of 30 feet or more. At the middle of the span, the vine cleared the ground by 18 inches and, for most of its length, it was six inches in diameter. I was reminded of the fact these are some of the largest lianas in the world. However, measuring them is no easy task. Getting up close to where the leaves are in the winding branches, it was nearly impossible not to get trapped. Many times, I had to carefully remove the claw-like hooks from my clothing to get out. And where they lace in and out of the forest canopy above, the vines are most difficult to follow. The hooks are more numerous at the very ends of the vines where they become thinnest and their stems begin to coil. From a distance, they give the ends of the vine the uncanny appearance of razor wire.

The vine was like some giant prehistoric snake. It was half submerged in the ground for at least 10 feet before it made the turn upwards. Along its sides on the ground I found secondary roots. Like legs on an old lizard, they serve as anchors to secure the massive weight of the stalk as it rises upward in its quest for light. Sprouting up out of the imbedded part along the ground, there were new growths, and at the base of the vine I found several roots extending in different directions.

Near the bottom of the vine, there was about 12 feet of bark missing. It was clear that someone had vandalized the vine. The fact they had left anything may offer a clue to their identity. It was more than enough for me to keep the location of the vine and the old plantation out of this book.

Guisella remembered there were many more vines in the area when she was young. I commented that perhaps local deforestation, to make way for more cultivated crops, had gradually reduced the amount of available moisture in the area.[150]

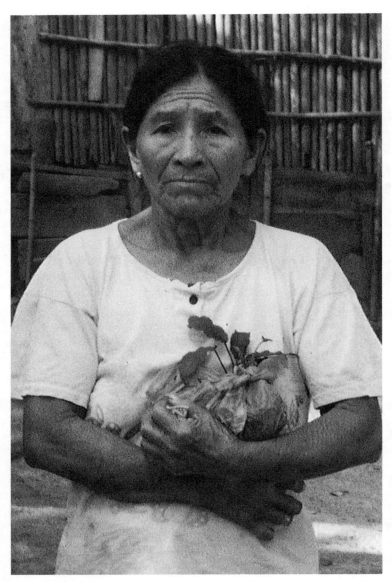

Elena, who told Brell about the use of cat's claw as a contraceptive.

Promise to Elena

The next morning I bid my guides a safe journey back to Lima where they had business to attend to. My new guides, the Brells, also had very busy lives and were most generous in the amount of time they shared.

After relating what Whitworth could recall about his expedition, Guisella's mother was able to name the key people involved. There was an Asháninka couple who were close friends of the family and had helped them during the war. At Brell's suggestion, the husband was recruited as Whitworth's guide. Since the wife was still living in the area, we decided to locate her for an interview. Her name was Elena. Elfriede recalled that Elena's first husband had saved Whitworth and his crew from death when their canoes capsized in a particularly treacherous piece of river. Her husband had died shortly after the expedition.[150]

Finding Elena took some time. There was no house along the road and no sign or street number to indicate anyone had ever lived in the area. Finally, Elfriede found the spot by looking for a certain point along the river. It was a trick she learned as a child when Elena and Elfriede played together as children. As soon as we could see a path, two barking dogs came rushing out to stop us. One looked fed and the other emaciated. While the dogs sniffed me over, a leaping monkey howled at me from the tree tops. From their thoughtful stares, I concluded that my odor was entirely alien.

Elfriede went in to lessen the shock the rest of us would surely make upon Elena. About half an hour later the signal came for us to enter. We climbed up a steep path that turned into the forest. Ahead of us we could see a portal made of twigs that required us to stoop to get through. The path curved towards a clearing where, in the center, a few wooden benches were arranged beside a fire pit. Elena, now 70 years old, came out to greet us. Elfriede told me when she contacted her 10 years ago Elena looked exactly the same.

Her house was made of wooden slats that rarely met. On the dirt floor I saw two cats. One appeared normal and the other emaciated, just like the dogs. It soon became apparent why. Elena's only means of income was spread out before us on a slab of concrete: a few square yards of drying cacao beans destined for a factory to make chocolate. Her second husband was very old and sick and had been taken to a hospital in Tarma, which was a great distance away. She was sad she couldn't afford to visit him more often and was now much poorer without him.[150,151]

Elena picked oranges from the trees behind us as a large brown bird glided overhead. Having quenched our thirst, we started the interview. She began by telling me that Arturo had always been interested in the medicinal plants that his workers used to keep themselves well. He collected information about medicinal plants for many years. It was another of his great many interests in the region. Arturo also learned to speak the language of his Indian workers and this opened the way to their knowledge. Elena recalled a man named Whitworth and another named Yates who came on an expedition. She was proud to tell me that her first husband saved their lives on the river and I felt fortunate to be able to tell her Whitworth had never forgotten.[151] He was grateful to this day.[5]

When I finally got around to the subject of cat's claw, Elena explained she had once mentioned a plant to Arturo that was used to prevent pregnancies. It was a vine the women crushed or pulverized to extract a liquid. I inquired about how much they had to take. Her fingers showed an amount of about one cup by our measurements. From further inquiries she explained the vine was only effective as a contraceptive when taken during the period of menstruation. Elena seemed very insistent the vine had to be used when fresh or it wouldn't be effective as a contraceptive. Guisella reminded me that Elena's memory was probably not what it used to be and we concluded what Elena was referring to was the root.[151] As for when to take the root, Brell had indicated the opposite: immediately following the menstrual cycle and in very high doses.[152]

I asked whether there was anything else she wanted to tell me. Elena said there was and then paused. She emphasized her message with one of her sturdy old hands gently raised in a fist. Like a judge's gavel, her hand came down to rest in the other as she spoke in a tone of warning: "If uña de gato ever becomes used as a contraceptive, it will only be right if due compensation is made to my people." Although I understood not a single word, her message scarcely needed translation. I grasped at once her message was somehow directed in homage to her ancestors, the Asháninka. As we parted, I promised to make her wishes known in my book.[151]

We left Elena what little money we could spare for food and to feed her animals. During the drive back to my hotel, and for the rest of the day, I found myself with little to say. All I could think about was Elena.

Two months later, Dr. Indacochea Herrera, president of the National College of Chemistry in Peru, announced that use of cat's claw as a contraceptive in Asháninka family planning should be scientifically investigated for national use. When I read that if cat's claw worked, Herrera also wanted to see the use of the vine as a contraceptive patented in Peru,[84] I had to wonder whether Elena knew that, inevitably, one day someone would prove cat's claw was effective.

A Grateful Shopkeeper

Nearing the end of another long day in the heat, I wanted only to have a shower, count my insect bites, and sleep. But as my impatient fate would have it, opportunity waited nearby. I learned that in a small store a few blocks from my hotel there was a woman who knew Brell when she was young. She wanted to tell us about the time that Arturo had helped her 23 years ago.

After a casual introduction, the shopkeeper agreed to a short interview, as soon as she attended her customers. She was about 40 years old and didn't mind discussing something so personal, if it would help. She began by telling us that at a time when most women marry, she was greatly troubled with recurring cysts. They grew around her breasts and upper torso and were about the size of grapes. Doctors operated on her twice and still the cysts returned. Friends referred her to people who knew Brell and soon a little bottle of extract became hers to try. She took the extract daily, only a few drops in juice or milk, three times a day for five months. The cysts disappeared and never returned. The sincerity of her thanks to the Brells for Arturo's kindness so long ago was touching. It was another reminder of the way people solved their struggles together in this frontier.

Midnight Express

Around midnight on my way back to the hotel, I spotted an eight-ton truck loaded with bundles of long strips of bark that I recognized instantly. I raced down the street to catch a gang of hurried workers before they could unload. I managed to get two pictures before I was abruptly told to stop. A young woman who spoke perfect English wanted to know who I was, what I was doing in Peru, and more. I had the same questions for her. Once I assured her I was not from a newspaper or someone else in "the business," she explained the bark was headed for Lima and then destined for Europe. In under 30 minutes, a team of men had thrown the entire load to the top of a bus. They suggested if I wanted to take pictures of cat's claw I should go to Puerto Bermúdez, a little spot on the map that today might also be called *Puerto Uña de Gato*. I recalled the road built to this place was supervised by Oscar Schuler, the son of the sawmill owner who had lung cancer and lived after taking Brell's extract. Puerto Bermúdez is where most of the bark in the region is brought for transport over the Andes to Lima. I had seen photos in the Peruvian press where bails the size of pickup trucks sat along the roadsides. I wondered just how many people collecting cat's claw had the necessary licences and permits. The Ministry of Agriculture also requires harvesters to plant new vines wherever they are cut or removed. Reassuring as that might be, I planned to discuss the matter of ecology with experts when I returned to Lima.

The Doctor from Lima

By the third day in Chanchamayo, word came that the mysterious doctor from Lima whom Whitworth had contacted had finally been located. He was visiting old friends in the town of La Merced, less than half a mile from my hotel. For the two of us to be in the same area during the same week in Peru, and in a place he visited only once a year, was truly uncanny. When finally we tracked him down he was at the mayor's house. It was only then that I learned his name: Dr. Manases Fernandez Lancho.

Dr. Fernandez had been a professor of biology in the School of Medicine at San Marcos University in Lima. In the early 1950s, he received a medal for vaccinating 13,000 people at risk of contracting yellow fever in Chanchamayo. The outbreak was so rampant that no other doctor in Peru dared go in. Shortly after his departure, representatives from the area journeyed to Lima to convince him to leave his teaching post and return, if only for a year. He ended up staying 11 years, founded the local Rotary Club in 1953, and recruited Brell and a few of his friends as members from the town of San Ramón.[153]

Dr. Fernandez thought for awhile, to refresh his memory of a time so long ago. I kept my questions for later. After a few rounds of freshly squeezed orange juice, we got around to the time Whitworth had set out on his expedition.

There was a Mr. Reiter who, for five years, lived with a group of Asháninka women. Professor Whitworth reached

Dr. Fernandez through a contact in the U.S. who hoped he could put them in touch with a guide. When Whitworth explained he wanted to study Ashâninka culture, Dr. Fernandez wrote Brell to find Mr. Reiter, since he would be an excellent guide.[153] The Brells still had the letter that Fernandez wrote to Arturo in May, 1964. The letter asks a favor of Brell to act as translator and to put Whitworth and his scientific mission in touch with Brell's cousin, Samuel Reiter. Whitworth was trying to reach a place called Pampa Michi. His team would be staying there a few days and since Brell's cousin was the "cacique" (minor chief) of the Ashâninkas in the area of the Perené River, he could be of great assistance.[154] We began to piece together a clearer picture of the events over another glass of fresh orange juice.[153]

Brell's work with medicinal plants was something Whitworth became fascinated with only after his experiences with Reiter and the Ashâninka,[153] which for Whitworth was, by all accounts, an incredible time.[5,155] It was on a second trip to the Indian villages that Brell had come along, but only to further his ongoing research.[5,153] Fernandez explained Brell had just returned from a visit to Germany in 1965 and had joked with him about how he spent some time studying medicine. I recalled Brell was, after all, a schoolteacher and Dr. Fernandez was the most respected physician in the area. What Dr. Fernandez didn't know was how serious Brell was in his studies of medicinal plants. When an article about Brell's formulas appeared in a Lima newspaper in 1974, he thought Brell had again succeeded in pulling everyone's leg. The article was about the owner of a sawmill in La Merced who recovered from lung cancer after taking an extract from Brell along with radiation treatments.[153]

The good doctor had a keen memory and so much fascinating history to tell, I could have listened to him for days. After drinking more of the local orange juice we parted hoping to meet again. I promised to send a copy of my book and to get in touch the next time I was in Peru.

Interview with Angel

The Brells and I traveled by bus from La Merced to the town of San Ramón in the hope of finding one of Arturo's oldest and dearest friends, a man named Angel Luna. Guisella only met him as a child, so we didn't know what to expect. The journey was especially beautiful. The sunlight seemed to bring out the full color of the foliage that day, which for me was an endless source of distraction, even from the window of a racing bus. I was amazed to see purple orchids growing straight out of dirt cliffs. Guisella mentioned they were unfortunately part of an illegal harvest in the area. The orchids were now being sold for export under the guise of "cultivated" plants from Peru.

We were extremely lucky to find Angel Luna at the same address Elfriede had kept for years. Angel lived in a tidy little house with a narrow brick passage that lead to a small open garden. After the dust and traffic nearby, it was like walking into another world. Lush ornamentals and fruit trees surrounded a soft carpet of deep green lawn bordered with select flowers and ferns. It was a place of peace filled with botanical curiosities. We settled into the dining room at a large wood table. Luna began to tell me about the days when Brell had begun his quest for cat's claw and the herbs he would finally use in combination.

Sometime in the early 1960s, Brell explored a rugged area of Peru known as the Gran Pajonal. Commonly regarded as a wild no-man's land, the Gran Pajonal lies northeast of San Ramón between the rivers Perené and Tambo in the south, the river Pachitea in the west, and the Ucayali River in the east. Here, the rivers run so wildly they are too dangerous to navigate. Based on the local climate, Brell thought cat's claw would probably grow very well in the Gran Pajonal. He also believed an immense number of varieties might occur here, especially at elevations of 3200-5000 feet, where he said the best and largest vines grew.[155]

When Luna explored the area after Brell, he tried to inquire about uses of the vine by conversing with the local Asháninkas. But on this matter he found they were very secretive. Luna wanted to know what uses they might make of the root bark since this was the part of the vine Brell believed was the most active. Luna tricked them using a method that all the best ethnobotanists employ. He simply dug up one of the roots and waited for the Indians to give him their reaction. They told him they couldn't understand why he wanted the root when the stalk bark was so much easier to obtain. To Luna that indicated they knew something about the vine after all. He eventually learned that the Asháninkas of the Gran Pajonal used the vine as a contraceptive, although it wasn't used alone. Some other plant, a member of the Liliaceae family which he never did learn, was combined with it. Brell had told Luna that it was the plant the Indians used more widely as a contraceptive in Peru. However, Brell insisted the Indians really didn't make much use of contraceptive plants. They were only taken to prevent having children from other tribes, such as when women were taken captive during wars and disputes.[155]

Luna found the Indians used a method of combining three or more plants. He also mentioned chuchuhuasi, a subject I looked into before my trip (see appendix). It was one of the plants the Indians combined with cat's claw, a fact that Brell had also noticed. Brell thought the two plants were similar in action and were both powerful anti-inflammatories. I reminded him I didn't want to learn Brell's formulas and I thought he was beginning to tell me too much. But he assured me the secrets of Brell's formulas were not known to him, either.[155]

I was curious to know what he could tell me about Brell's observations from the many people who had used his formulas. As Brell explained to Luna, the way they worked was essentially by increasing the body's defenses. He believed they slowed the aging process, improved the quality of the skin and hair, caused liver spots to vanish, and improved the vision. Luna told me he could personally attest to benefiting from cat's claw for his rheumatism. He explained he had been taking the liquid

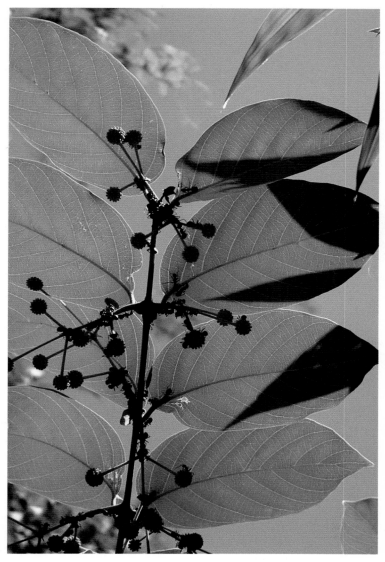

K. Jones, 1995

1. The top of cat's claw (Uncaria tomentosa (Willd.) DC) preparing to bloom. Chanchamayo Valley, Peru.

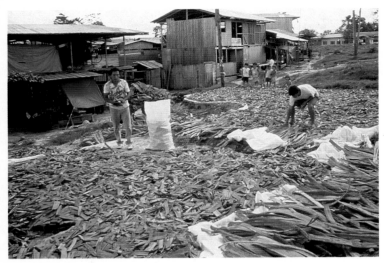

Carlos Guillén, 1995

2. Workers bagging the sun-dried inner bark of cat's claw in Pucalpa, Peru.

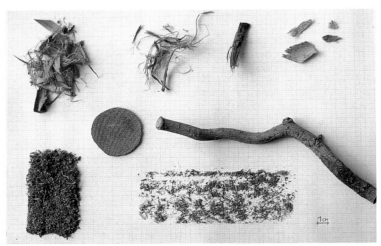

Courtesy of Immodal Pharmak, Volders, Austria

3. Root parts of *Uncaria tomentosa*. Top line (left to right): shavings of inner bark, a piece of bark, and wood shavings. Second line: cross section of large root; piece of root. Bottom line: finely cut root for preparing medicinal tea.

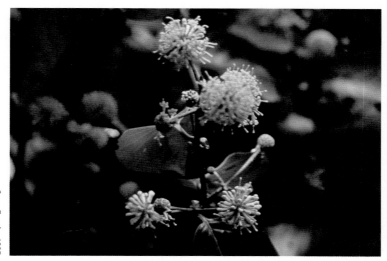

Cesar Zavala, 1995

4. *Uncaria tomentosa* in bloom.

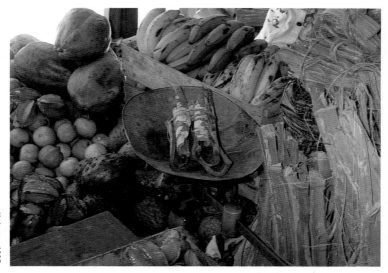

K. Jones, 1995

5. Weighing out some chuchuhuasi in the marketplace of La Merced. Note the stalk bark of cat's claw on the right.

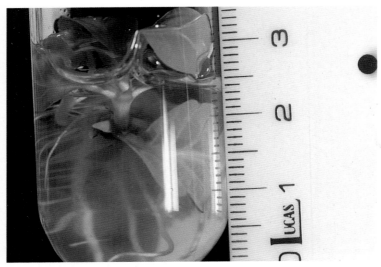

6. Cat's claw grown from leaf in a test tube (*in vitro*).

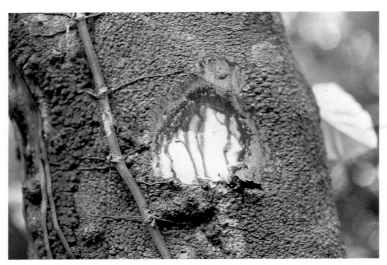

7. The healing sap of a wounded sangre de drago tree
(Croton lechleri L.).

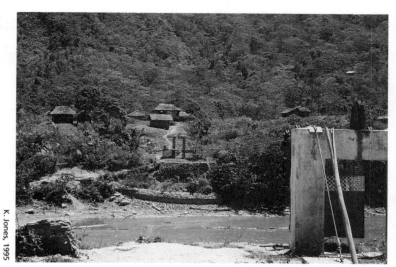

River dwellings along the road to Pinchanaki.

K. Jones, 1995

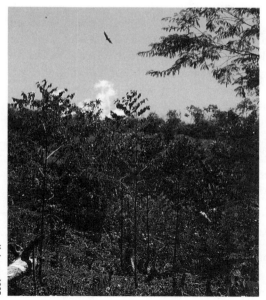

An experimental field of uña de gato (*Uncaria tomentosa*) near Pichanaki, Peru.

K. Jones, 1995

extract he makes himself for many years now and his rheumatism was well under control. I noted he was in his seventies and didn't look a day over 50, despite the fact he was also a heavy smoker. Luna makes his extract by taking the root bark and allowing it to soak in 42% sugar cane alcohol for a period of three to four hours. He takes three to four drops, with liquids, three times a day. Luna recalled Brell used a similar method. He steeped the bark in a mixture of 50% boiled water and 50% brandy and thought this was the best way to make the extract. He also insisted certain roots were better than others and told Luna that vines growing in shadier areas were superior.[155]

Luna didn't know about any scientific work Brell might have done, but was certain he had sent cat's claw to Austria for testing between 1966 and 1968. The results showed the presence of at least five alkaloids and some steroidal or hormonal compounds which I deduced must have been sterols.[155]

I wondered whether Brell had ever told him about the Whitworth expedition. He told me Brell hadn't spoken very much about it, but he did recall Brell saying he had watched Whitworth take hallucinogenic plants with the shamans, an experience Brell declined. Angel laughed when I told him Whitworth was a much braver explorer than I had thought.[155]

Now I saw why Whitworth could lay claim to having been shown so much by the Indians. He was probably one of the few foreigners with whom the shamans he met had ever shared their hallucinogens. And since these are the kinds of plants that shamans sometimes take to diagnose and to prescribe medicines for their patients, it was as if Whitworth had been allowed a peek into their pharmacy.

Luna had given me much to ponder. I was especially curious about the matter of micro-climate and Brell's insistence that cat's claw collected from shadier areas worked best.[155] It was Keplinger who reported the local Indians recognized three vari-

eties of cat's claw in central Peru. Traditionally distinguished by
the color of the freshly cut vine, there was a dark red, a yellow-
brown, and a white-gray variety. The red one seems to prefer a
warm and moist climate, whereas the white-gray cat's claw
appears to prefer a cool and dry area. The yellow-brown variety occurs in areas that are somewhere between a moist and
warm climate and a cool and dry one. He added that as far as
contents of oxindole alkaloids are concerned, any correlation to
climate or color has been impossible to establish.[101] The matter
was studied over 10 years ago by the Ludwig Maximilians
University in Munich. There was no way to tell what the alkaloid content would be from one year, one month, or even one
part of the vine to the next, whether in the leaves, root, or stalk
of any colored cat's claw.[95] (See appendix: Variable Levels of
Alkaloids.)

A Field of Uña de Gato

On my last day in Chanchamayo, I ventured out much far-
ther than I had gone before. Guisella and I hoped to visit a
place where there was an experimental plot of cultivated cat's
claw. On the way, we passed orange and olive groves that grew
in neat rows up from the Perené River below. In some places
they stretched a mile or more. Further out, we passed small villages of Asháninkas. I watched Indians fishing the river using
traditional methods of net and spear. Apart from farm trucks,
the main means of transport was by canoe and what few buildings I could see were entirely made of thatched palms and
wood beams.

Several miles further along the dusty old road, any passing
vehicles became scarce. As we rounded another bend, we saw a
produce truck detained beside a troop transporter with 20 mm
machine-guns on top. Without warning, two Sinchi paratroop-
ers with automatic rifles lunged out in front of us. After check-
ing our papers, they asked whether we had been stopped by

anyone else along the road. We were happy to say we had not and they allowed us to drive on. Their presence was reassuring because this far out terrorists were still active in the area.

We finally reached our destination past the town of Pichanaki. But there wasn't as much to see as we had hoped. The half acre or so of planted vines was obviously experimental. In the open and without any shade, many of the vines produced leaves with what looked like blisters. They appeared so diseased I commented, "These uña de gato may *need* uña de gato." The young vines showed they had first grown up like bushes and had become like small trees. When they reached a height of about nine feet, their tops arched down towards the ground or any nearby tree that would support them.

Through a translator, I spoke with some of the local Asháninka. I asked them what part of the vine was being harvested here. It was the root, but personally they never used that part of cat's claw because then their source of bark would be gone. The Indians didn't have a seedling farm to replace the vines, so using the root just wasn't practical. Nearby, we were told there were much larger plantation sites of cat's claw we could visit, but not today. The caretaker was away and would not return until late that night.

The intense heat of the day was ending and, since one of the members of our little expedition risked severe shock from an allergic reaction to insect bites, I thanked the Indians for their courtesy and we left before nightfall.

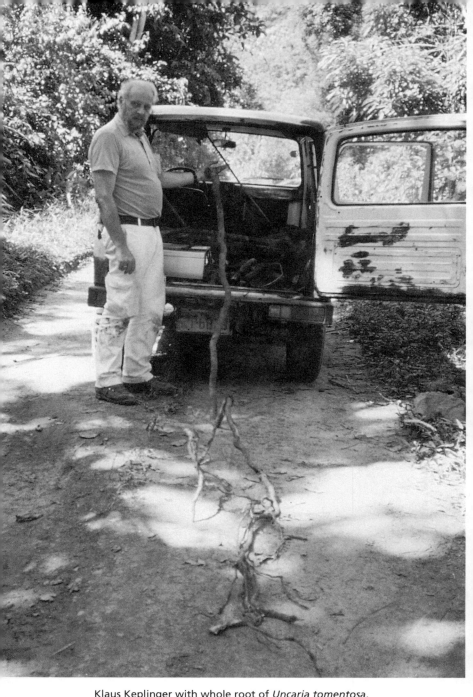

Klaus Keplinger with whole root of *Uncaria tomentosa*.

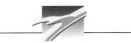

IV.
Research in Peru

I boarded a bus for the long trip back to Lima. It was equipped with a television monitor for the day's movie, another Ninja thriller. But the scenery kept me glued to the window all the way. From the height of the bus, I saw the journey across the Andes was far more dangerous than I had first thought. Looking back, the Andean highway was the most treacherous part of my entire trip. However, the scenery was so stunning that the danger seemed trivial.

Along much of the winding highway, mountain gorges a yard or so from the pavement drop at least a 3000 feet down. Except for a few guard rails here and there, and thin ones at that, nothing would stop a vehicle from plunging over the side. A V-shaped cement ditch that runs along many of the steeper parts of the road presents another source of danger. One wheel entering the ditch can force the rest of the vehicle to be dragged into the rock face of the road. An entire side of one unlucky bus I noticed was mangled like a beer can. What passengers remained lined up in the cold, waiting for another bus to come along. Another mile or so down I gasped at the remains of a transport truck. After plunging 100 feet or more to the next level of the road, the entire cab was flattened to the thickness of a pizza box. Apparently the load of hardwood logs it was carrying had followed the driver's section on the way down.

As soon as my bus entered the outskirts of Lima, it was stopped by soldiers at the district border. Outside, the air was chilly. Some passengers, especially the poor, were removed for questioning. My passport was taken and returned in half an hour. It was another routine check for terrorists trying to enter the city. The majority of terrorists in Peru have been captured, but some remain at large.

I awoke the next day to gray skies and a cold room. It was still winter in Lima. I learned over lunch with colleagues that a bus on the way from San Ramón to Satipo had been stopped, unloaded, and blown up during the week I was in the area. I was told if the terrorists had been members of the Sendero Luminoso, or Shining Path, the bus would have been blown up *with* the passengers onboard. I was later informed that recent terrorist activities around the cat's claw plantation where I had visited with the Brells precluded my safe return in the near future. Yet no one I met in Chanchamayo seemed especially concerned. The locals resign themselves to a common saying: Terrorists are like the rain.

The Department of Chemistry

One of my first appointments in Lima was with Professor Olga Lock de Ugaz, coordinator of the Department of Chemistry at the Pontificia Universidad Católica del Peru. As we discussed the needs for new research of cat's claw, she informed me that a three-year phytochemical study was now well underway. Findings would not be revealed until publication. However, she was willing to answer my questions regarding the amount of tannins in cat's claw. Studies found the inner stalk bark contained about 20% tannins,[156] or 200 mg/gram, which is a fairly high amount.

Dr. Lock's colleagues at the university were also looking into the area of culturing the root. Their goal is to eventually find a way to produce the root in tanks filled with the nutrients necessary to produce consistent material on a large scale.[156] The potential advantages of this technology are enormous. Not only could levels of active constituents be provided more consistently, the rain forests could be left intact because the natural root, stalk, or leaves could be grown almost anywhere, continuously.[157] It is also anticipated a significant amount of growing time could be saved by providing harvesting sites with the cultured vines once they become acclimatized in greenhouses. Dr. Lock agreed there were many other medicinal plants to which this *in vitro* (in glass) technology could be applied.[156]

In fact, growing *Uncaria* leaves in culture had already been accomplished five years ago at the National University of Singapore.[158] And at the National Agrarian University of Molina in Lima, others claimed success in developing *in vitro* micropropagation techniques with *Uncaria tomentosa* and *U. guianensis* from seeds.[159] Ostensibly, their next step could be to grow the root *in vitro*.

We discussed several ideas for future activity studies of cat's claw and hoped to meet again.[156] Just as I was about to leave, she kindly presented me with her most recent review of activity studies on cat's claw, now a cherished memento of my visit.[160]

The Ministry of Health

The following day, I had an appointment at the Ministry of Health at the National Institute of Traditional Medicine of Peru—another sadly under-funded effort to improve a nation's health by increasing awareness of medicinal plants. I met with the chairman, the respected Peruvian neurologist Dr. Fernando Cabieses, a researcher in the field of ethnopharmacology and a recognized authority on the subject of cat's claw. He agreed the whole subject needed more research. Many of the claims people were making about the vine were as yet unfounded by science. Against AIDS, for example, he explained that any studies in Peru were preliminary and that contrary to the optimism conveyed in the Peruvian press, so far the results were inconclusive.[161]

He asked me what kinds of studies I thought were needed at

this point. My reply was that traditional uses of the vine by the Indians of Peru were still high on my list and I thought the contraceptive use needed further study. We hoped to talk again and parted after sharing some of the more humorous sides of medicinal plant research.[161]

Cat's claw had been used to treat AIDS in Europe since the mid-1980s.

I left the interview thinking about the difficult problem of AIDS. I had been gathering articles on the subject for some time. Cat's claw had been used to treat AIDS in Europe since the mid-1980s. The idea of applying cat's claw in AIDS started in Austria in 1984, and the Peruvian press had been emphasizing the subject ever since.[159,160] Yet, it was obvious from my interview with Cabieses that no one in Peru was certain whether or not cat's claw was of any benefit to people with AIDS.

For most medical scientists an affordable treatment for AIDS is only a dream. If AIDS continues its spread at current rates of incidence, many patients in poorer countries will go without any treatment. The present cost of the drugs alone would bankrupt entire countries. The use of a medicinal plant that could be grown throughout most of the tropics would be a highly welcomed development. If it were only to provide symptomatic relief and were to prolong life, such a product would still be a lot cheaper than the drugs currently used to treat AIDS — drugs that don't do much more.

To think millions of AIDS patients are going to be able to afford a drug like AZT (zidovudine), or one equally expensive, is naive at best. For example, a new combination treatment, AZT plus ddI (didanosine) or ddC (dideoxycytidine), was recently found to extend the life of AIDS patients by over two years. But the cost is equal to what a doctor in Uganda makes in 10 years[164] and when you add the growing problem of heterosexual transmission — currently responsible for 75% of cases worldwide — the 8-10 million people currently infected are bound to become a comparatively small number.[165]

AIDS Research

So what does anyone really know about the effect of cat's claw with regard to AIDS? So far, not as much as one might hope, at least not in any published reports. The inconclusive results that Cabieses referred to concern a small number of patients who were monitored for a period of three months at a hospital in Lima. There were no "adverse effects."[166] We also discussed the excitement in Peru about a group of patients in Iquitos who took cat's claw and appeared to be living symptom-free.[161]

Dr. Roberto Inchaustegui Gonzales, Head of the Committee of Transmissible Diseases and AIDS at the Hospital of the Peruvian Institute of Social Security in Iquitos, presented a report on his preliminary findings in February 1993. His patients had shown positive readings for the disease in the ELISA test, but not conclusively in other tests. Five patients who had been having unprotected sex with multiple partners showed symptoms associated with AIDS, such as swollen lymph nodes, chronic diarrhea, *Herpes zoster*, and pneumonia. They were given cat's claw tea (*U. tomentosa* and *U. guianensis*) — 1/4 cup divided in three doses every eight hours. One patient, who also had hemorrhagic tuberculosis and was spitting up blood, was given an herb called "sacha jergón," which was added at the same daily dose. When after six months tests showed a negative reading for HIV, the rest of the patients were put on the same formula. Later, their readings were also negative for the virus.[167-169] However, when some of these patients were given more accurate tests (ELISA and Western blot), readings showed they were still HIV-positive.[169]

The herb that Dr. Inchaustegui added to his formula, sacha jergón (*Dracontium peruvianum*),[168] is a tuberous plant with snake-like scales. The tubers of *Dracontium* species are used in the Amazon to make a flour for food. The flour is also used to treat asthma and, made into a paste, it serves as a plaster which is applied directly on snake bites.[170,171]

Meanwhile, the Peruvian press reports that in Austria physicians monitoring AIDS patients taking a proprietary root product of *Uncaria tomentosa* have reported that in five years their subjects have shown practically no symptoms. In 1992, they started to monitor a group taking AZT as well. Experiments in rabbits showed a definite increase in CD4 lymphocytes (helper T-cells) following injections of the root extract. Since CD4 cells are among the main immune cells destroyed by HIV, it is now hoped cat's claw will increase the life-span of AIDS patients, as well as reducing the side-effects of AIDS drugs, such as AZT.[172]

AIDS patients in Austria and Germany have been taking standardized root products of cat's claw for the last 10 years. Some have reported remission of their symptoms, even of a skin cancer (Kaposi's sarcoma)[162] common in AIDS which is caused by human Herpes virus 8.[173,174] Although a modest amount of antiviral activity has been found in quinovic acid glycosides from the root bark (*U. tomentosa*), the doses required bordered on toxic amounts and the viruses inhibited (vesicular stomatitis virus and rhinovirus) were not HIV.[175] The main benefits to AIDS patients would be largely the result of other components, such as pentacyclic oxindole alkaloids.

An observational study of AIDS patients in Europe taking root extracts of cat's claw has been running for many years. Recent findings are based on a substance called IMM-207, which is composed of six pentacyclic alkaloids contained in a standardized cat's claw root extract. In 1992, Dr. Ursula Keplinger, whose father is Klaus Keplinger, presented clinical results with this preparation at the AIDS Congress in Zurich, Switzerland,[176] and in 1993 at the 4th Austrian AIDS Congress in Vienna.[177] Results involving 10 female and 34 male AIDS patients have since been updated to 1994.[7] The following is a brief summary of what the results have shown:

The majority of the patients received the standardized extract powder in capsules, and 36 received a daily dose of 20 milligrams. The remainder of the patients took daily doses of extract of not more than 60 milligrams. Of the total cases, 15 took AZT as well, while the other 23 took only the root extract. Those patients who showed symptoms prior to taking the extract became free of symptoms, including recurrent *Herpes simplex* and vaginal and oral fungal infections.[7]

The patients who had CD4 lymphocyte counts of 200-500 (CDC 2) fared the best. Their CD4 cells increased by significant amounts for the first year of therapy and the increase persisted for the first three years. The fact that patients continued to show stable CD4 cell counts for as long as four and five years after beginning to receive the root extract is remarkable. Yet "none of the patients documented for that period showed a decline to less than 200," which would have placed them in the next level of AIDS progression (CDC 3). Their p24 antigen level (used as a marker for HIV) declined and their B-cell (B-lymphocyte) counts increased. The CDC 2 patients taking both AZT and the extract showed the same improvement in their CD4 cell counts by the end of the first six months as those on the extract alone.[7]

If the extract now being studied in Europe proves to be as good as AZT, as well as less toxic, you can be sure the entire world will know. I expect in a few more years we will finally see the results of new studies with the extract in AIDS and can then read some judgments. Until then, there is good cause for hope.

One for the Animals

While reading the material given to me by Professor Ugaz, I noticed she cited the work of a Peruvian veterinarian named Dr. Victor Humberto Ruiz.[160] In May 1994, Dr. Ruiz had impressed Cabieses with his findings at a meeting on cat's claw sponsored by the World Health Organization in Geneva.[161] Dr. Ruiz had performed one of the most intriguing studies of the vine to date,[178] and yet, no one I knew had even heard of the man. I was determined to locate him.

The next day I headed for his department at the University of San Marcos. His assistant, Dr. Victor Fernandez, was just finishing with a patient in surgery. He regretted to inform me that Dr. Ruiz had passed away in 1994. Dr. Fernandez, Chief of the Laboratory of Pharmacology and Toxicology, now carries on where his professor left off. In one corner of his office, there was a large stack of bark strips. They were the same kind of dried inner stalk bark I had seen in the marketplaces of Chanchamayo. Dr. Fernandez informed me this cat's claw had come from the Shipibo Indians in eastern Peru near Pucallpa. He then graciously agreed to an interview.[179]

We began by reviewing the kinds of cases he had treated and the preparations he used. In most cases he was treating dogs with an injectable preparation (50% alcohol/water) made by a process that removed the tannins which are potentially lethal when injected intravenously. The solution was autoclaved for sterility and usually given once a day, 3 cc at a time. Recently, he had treated a boxer for tumors in the mouth and forepaws. The treatment required four months and was successful.[179]

He showed me a diary of cases and their outcomes. I saw that respiratory disorders were treated in one week and the injections were also used to treat lymphoma, dermatitis, and distemper. A vaccine is available for distemper, but not all dogs are vaccinated in Peru. The disease can be severe in the last stages with 30 or 40 convulsions a day. Yet, even in these cases, he had success. After one injection he saw the convulsions reduced in frequency to one or two a day. The convulsions stopped on the third day of treatment. He had a small dog in his clinic who had distemper despite the available vaccine. The dog had received one injection of the extract every 24 hours and was now doing very well. An akita he had recently treated required four injections. The dog was fine and, like the others, it would not have to be destroyed.[179]

Dr. Fernandez went on to describe the case of a dog who was operated on for a fractured leg. The metal pin that had been inserted to hold the dog's bones together was much too big and caused an open and infected wound nearly 8 inches long. He applied an ointment he had formulated with cat's claw and the wound was then covered and bound with gauze and tape. The size of the wound had reduced by 50% after three weeks.[179]

Cat's claw was just one of several medicinal plants that Dr. Fernandez had been experimenting with. We discussed some of his work in developing ointments for vitiligo in humans and for difficult fungal infections. His preliminary results were most encouraging and provide further evidence of the great potential of the medicinal flora of Peru.[179]

The Peruvian pioneer of cat's claw in veterinary medicine was Dr. Fernandez's professor, Dr. Humberto Ruiz Urbina (1918-1994). Dr. Ruiz received his doctorate in veterinarian medicine at the University of Texas and a further degree in pharmacology at the University of Michigan. Among his many honored positions and achievements, Dr. Ruiz was founder and professor of the Faculty of Veterinarian Medicine at the National University Mayor de San Marcos, and he served as President of the Association of Veterinarian Physicians of Peru.[180] Dr. Ruiz spoke about his results at a World Health Organization meeting on cat's claw held in Switzerland, in May 1994. Owing to his death, it is unlikely that his results will be published in the near future, if at all. Therefore, the following summary, with comments on the findings he presented in Geneva, may serve to preserve the honor due Dr. Ruiz as a pioneer in this field.

Dr. Ruiz used various preparations of cat's claw: a tea made by steeping the inner stalk bark in hot water, the traditional bark decoction made by boiling the bark in water, finely powdered bark pulverized and encapsulated, bark extract powder (freeze-dried) in pill form,[178,181] a fluid extract (distillate), and a bark tincture (5 ml equivalent to one gram of bark powder).[182] From 1990 to 1994, he experimented with cat's claw in treating 53 cats and 135 dogs for a wide range of problems (see table), many of them difficult to treat by any means.

Those dogs given the bark lived two to three years longer than untreated dogs.

Nearly half the cats and over a quarter of the dogs he treated with the bark had cancer of the mammary glands. Dr. Ruiz reported that all the preparations he used had stopped the tumors from growing and decreased their size by 20%. From the start of treatment, the cats lived three to four years longer than untreated cats with mammary tumors. Those dogs given the bark lived two to three years longer than untreated dogs. He noted mammary tumors generally appear at around the age of 10 in these animals. Why tumors occur at all in cats and dogs was still being investigated.[181,182]

Some of the dogs he treated lived past the age of 16. Some of the cats he treated with the bark alone lived to the age of 15, which was longer than cats treated with surgery plus cat's claw who lived for only one more year — still, a year more than most cats lived with surgery alone.[178]

Dr. Ruiz treated another 10 cats and 20 dogs for inflammation and allergic reactions of the skin, which were largely due to insect bites, especially from fleas. The treatment with cat's claw usually lasted one to three months, or until the animals recuperated. He noted that they all showed "new and soft fur."[178,182]

As part of his presentation in Geneva, Dr. Ruiz made note of the fact there were other causes of allergic reactions in dogs and cats in Peru, besides flea bites. The digestion of insects, including bees and flies, and foods that ferment in the digestive tract, such as sweet potatoes and oat meal, were also known to cause allergic reactions that created itching. Animals that rubbed their skin against the ground or on walls to relieve the itching developed hair loss and lesions. Given the dusty and dirty conditions in Lima, Dr. Ruiz observed that dermatitis in cats and dogs was especially common.[178,182] The incidence of infected lesions (pioderma) in the cat and dog population of Lima would naturally be higher, especially in those affected with allergic reactions of the skin.

Veterinary Applications of Cat's Claw

(University Mayor de San Marcos, Lima, 1990-94).[182]

Allergic Reactions to Insect Bites (hair loss, itching)
Geriatria (dull coat, hair loss, lethargy, poor skin)
Inflammation (muscle, prostate, stomach)
Hemorrhoids (rectal)
Mammary Tumors
Osteoarthritis
Parvovirosis
Dermatitis
Spondilitis
Coxaplana
Seborrhea
Pioderma
Arthritis

Using a distilled preparation of the bark, Dr. Ruiz treated 15 dogs for parvovirus[182]—a highly contagious, highly resistant disease spread primarily by infected feces. The virus appeared in 1978 and soon traveled around the world. Diarrhea, vomiting, high fever, and listlessness are the main symptoms and severe infection is marked by shock and death. The best defense is vaccination, but, in Peru, not enough people take the precaution or can afford to pay for the vaccine. Ideally, vaccination should be started when dogs are still puppies and completed before the age of 12 weeks.[183]

The treatment with cat's claw was given in two daily doses of 10 ml per 10 kg of body weight. Ten of the dogs that Dr. Ruiz treated recovered. The other five were dead by the third day. He reported that the 10 who recovered continued to receive the distillate for 30 days.[182]

With the finely pulverized bark in capsules, Dr. Ruiz used a dosage of 250-300 mg for every 10 kg of body weight (25-30 mg/kg). The dosage was always "divided in two doses per day." The bark powder was prescribed to treat old cats and dogs who showed signs of osteoarthritis and symptoms of old age, such as pain, poor appetite, malaise, and no inclination to run or walk. Dr. Ruiz told his audience that, over a period of four years, he had treated 15 cats and 30 dogs with these symptoms; the cats all around age 12 and the dogs all about nine years old.[182] He reported new hair grew in as "a soft and brilliant fur, as it is in young animals."[178] He also noted their appetite returned and their pains decreased "progressively."[178,182]

The treatment of inflammatory conditions with cat's claw was performed in 22 dogs with a hereditary and very painful disease commonly known as hip dysplasia. Dr. Ruiz pointed out the disease also occurs in people, horses, rabbits, cats, and cattle. He found cat's claw provided "rapid relief of great pain"[178] and dogs recuperated from the disease following one to three months of treatment. Again, he used the capsules of finely powdered bark. Beyond what he witnessed as a pain-relieving/anti-inflammatory activity,[182] the pharmacological effects of cat's claw in hip dysplasia remain unknown.

Hip dysplasia starts when dogs are young. The hip joint forms abnormally and this, in turn, affects the development of normal bone growth and the way joints conform. The resulting abnormal distribution of weight upon joints leads to joint disease. Degenerated cartilage, atrophied muscles, ruptured ligaments, and abrasions on bones have all been found to characterize this condition. In 30% of dogs genetically susceptible to the condition, degenerated cartilage also occurs in other body parts, such as the shoulder, elbow, and vertebral joints.[184]

In people, hip dysplasia occurs in women in 80% of cases. This is likely due to laxity of joints caused by an abnormality in estrogen metabolism. When estrogen is given to normal puppies, it can cause hip dysplasia. However, puppies that already have the condition show normal levels of estrogen.[184]

Injections of a proprietary root extract have been applied in the treatment of cats with feline leukemia and feline immunodeficiency virus (FIV).

Although surgery is the preferred means of treatment, hip dysplasia is known to be managed with pain-killers and anti-inflammatory drugs. In young dogs, drug therapy alone has an estimated 72% chance of bringing pain and laxity of joints back to a functional, pain-free state after they reach 18 months old. The problem is most drugs cause unwanted side-effects.[185] With hip dysplasia, as indeed with any medical problem in your animal, discuss all the options available with your veterinarian. In many cases, it may be wise to seek a second and even a third opinion.

Inflammation of the vertebral discs or spondilitis, is another abnormality commonly found in dogs. During the same four-year pilot study, Dr. Ruiz treated 18 dogs with this problem. He described the condition as one that begins with severe pain in the vertebral column. Then the back shows increasing paralysis until the animal can only move by crawling. Dr. Ruiz confirmed the diagnosis by taking X-rays of the protruding intervertebral discs so as not to confuse the problem with fractured vertebra. Specifically, he was looking for lesions of the fibrotic ring. In some cases they appear torn, and in others, the ring is completely ruptured. He explained the usual treatment is painkillers and anti-inflammatory agents.[178,182] Dr. Ruiz prescribed the bark powder in the usual dose, "until the intense pain is controlled and the animal recuperates from its paralysis." Such a desirable result, he added, required "many weeks."[182]

Veterinary experiments with cat's claw have also been underway in Austria. Injections of a proprietary root extract have been applied in the treatment of cats with feline leukemia and feline immunodeficiency virus (FIV). Dr. Ursula Keplinger presented the findings at the AIDS Congress in Vienna, Austria, in 1991. Intramuscular injections of a standardized root extract were given on the first, third, and fifth day of the treatment at a dose of 0.03 mg (in saline). The cats receiving the extract showed a disappearance of symptoms in 85% of cases. For the cats with leukemia, by the end of the twentieth week, 44% were free from the presence of the feline leukemia virus (FeLV) in their blood.[7] Since there are no treatments for either disease, these results offer hope that effective treatments might be at hand.

FIV was first reported in 1987. Estimates of the incidence of the disease in the U.S. vary from 1% to 7.4%. Thankfully, FIV doesn't infect people.[186] As with FIV, a vaccine is available for feline leukemia. Without the vaccine, an infected cat is expected to die. The virus that causes feline leukemia was found in 1964. Today, this is the major disease causing death in cats. Transmitted through feces, urine, and saliva, feline leukemia can easily be spread to unvaccinated cats. It is interesting to note that for about 40% of cats exposed to FeLV, their immune system will protect them against the virus and they will even develop immunity. For the other 60% of cats exposed to FeLV, half become carriers and the other half develop symptoms. The only treatment available has to be given two to three weeks following exposure, which is very difficult to determine. Moreover, the drug has side-effects and only stops the symptoms. The same drug (AZT) is used to treat AIDS.[187]

The Brell Papers

Peru can be like a friend who becomes easier to visit than to leave. The people, the old buildings, the marketplaces, and the many fascinating foods were just a few of the many distractions I just didn't have nearly enough time for. Over a pisco sour and a *resaca*, I consoled myself with the thought that there would always be other adventures waiting in this fascinating country, especially in the realm of medicinal plants.

A day before my departure, I had one last meeting with the Brells. As promised, they showed me a box full of letters, an archive of Arturo's ceaseless efforts to have his extracts studied scientifically. His notes were something Guisella had never bothered to go over and, two months later, she was still finding more of them.

A letter in the spring of 1970 captured the situation Whitworth faced in attempting to get Brell's extracts studied in the U.S. Brell had written concerning the progress of Mr. Schuler, to which Whitworth responded that even if one man's life had been prolonged, it would not bring needed recognition of "the herbs." Only adequate funding for tests, or the interest of the right people at the right time, would ever make a difference. But Brell was not to lose faith. In the hope of better days to come, Whitworth's wife enclosed a check for $100.00 for the completion of the Research Center.[188] There would be other checks from Whitworth, but Brell never cashed any of them.[189]

By the following spring, Whitworth had started a writing campaign. He assured Brell it wouldn't be long before Associated Press, United Press, the *San Francisco Chronicle*, Walter Cronkite at CBS, and other media sources would all know about Brell and cat's claw. Along with "documents," he enclosed a press release[190] on the progress Brell had been making in Peru. In 1971, the media learned that a medicinal plant brought from the jungles of Asháninka territory in the Perené River basin was being tested against cancer. Prepared as an extract by Arturo Brell of Chanchamayo, Peru, clinical tests were being conducted by a world-renowned cancer specialist, Dr. Miró-Quesada, Director General of the Peruvian National Institutes of Health. The extract was reportedly "effective" in volunteer patients with inoperable and incurable cancers of the bone, breast, and lung. Brell wanted to cultivate the plant with the idea of making the herb cheaper and more readily available for the masses. He was even suggesting the extract be made available as an additive for candy bars and soft drinks.[191]

Brell's historic letter to President Nixon in 1970 described the work accomplished to date.

The news release contained quotes from a letter that Brell sent to U.S. President Richard Nixon[192] at the suggestion of Whitworth.[193] Ironically, the letter arrived just nine months before Nixon officially declared "war on cancer" on December 23, 1971, as a Christmas gift to the American people.[194] Nixon responded. He requested the U.S. Embassy in Lima to reach Dr. Miró-Quesada and Brell, concerning the studies with cat's claw.[195] Sadly, in the long struggle to have cat's claw researched, that event was one of the rarer moments for optimism.

They were blocked at nearly every turn. Pharmaceutical companies wouldn't send equipment or staff. People they approached for donations grew reluctant. Members of the Cancer Society made themselves unavailable. And, while letters sent to U.S. senators were never answered, including Senator

Barry Goldwater, whose office refused even to acknowledge that a letter had been received, Whitworth wrote that when Brell sent word to President Nixon, however, "we got an immediate action."[191]

Brell's historic letter to President Nixon in 1970 described the work accomplished to date. He wrote about the case of Mr. Luis Schuler, "71 years old, lung cancer, non-operable, radiation treatment (cobalt bombardment) to the maximum tolerance without result, continuous cough," who, following 75 days on the extract, was found "restored to health." Brell noted Schuler became so well that he crossed the Andes at an altitude of 15,000 feet, "without oxygen." Other cases could be cited, he added, but a report he enclosed on the preliminary observations of Dr. Miró-Quesada in terminal cancer patients was more telling and, of course, more scientific. In closing, he stated, "I believe, Mr. President, that you can do something so that the research by myself and Dr. Whitworth and now by the Miró-Quesada group can be used for the benefit of humanity...and the rest of the world. I only wish to put this hope in your hands. For America and mankind."[192]

Poring over the letters that Whitworth wrote to Brell, I found they confirmed much of what he stated in his press release. To their credit, the Peruvian National Institutes of Health were extremely interested in Brell's work before interest was shown by Nixon. In November 1970, the Institute wrote Brell, stating, "given the importance of your findings in cures derived from traditional (folkloric) medical therapy... The Institute of National Health names you as a member of the investigative team for the Studies of Experimental Treatment of Cancer and other illnesses, that can be surveyed from the use of indigenous plants that you have furnished us with...and whatever work is published as a result of these investigations you will be a co-author."[8] The honor was furthered by a request from President Nixon the following year.[195]

At Nixon's urging, the U.S. National Cancer Institute (NCI) became involved in the summer of 1971. A letter from Robert

J. Avery, Jr. of the NCI was sent to Whitworth asking for a pound of the herb for testing. They also wanted to know the dosage used and "other details of its use."[195] Avery sent a letter to Dr. Anthony Donovan, Public Health Advisor for the Agency for International Development (AID), in Lima. He referred to something called "Karate-In," a name Quesada's group had given to a combination therapy consisting of chemotherapy and the "Brell C. H." extract,[196] the "C. H." meaning Chanchamayo.[189] According to Avery, the National Cancer Institute wanted to know about this, too:

"As for the polychemotherapeutic treatment of cancer called 'Karate-In'... Institute scientists believe it is quite possible it would be highly active against carcinomas. They would be interested in full case reports on the use of this drug on cancer patients if such are available."[196]

After treatment with Brell's extract, 10 infants had recuperated from leukemia. Some were still in remission four years later, but the research didn't last.

At this development, which was ostensibly a method of some merit—weakening tumors with chemotherapy and then boosting the immune system to kill them off—Brell became most disappointed. He wanted to see his extract tested by itself, not mixed up with something he felt was too toxic to the system. But that wish was too much to hope for, at least in his lifetime.[189]

Throughout 1971, interest in cat's claw and Brell's extract continued to grow. With promising contacts from the Peruvian Cancer Society, Dr. Eduardo Caceres, Director of the National Institute of Neoplastic Diseases in Lima, and from the American Cancer Society and the U.S. National Institutes of

Health, Whitworth was still optimistic.[197]

By the winter of 1971, the National Cancer Institute in the U.S. had received the requested sample of the vine and identified it as *Uncaria guianensis*.[198] But in Brell's papers, it appears that another three years passed before the results of the tests became known. They show up in a letter to one of Brell's many interested contacts, Dr. K. Jewers of the famous Tropical Products Institute in London, England. It was from Jonathan L. Hartwell, Head of the Natural Products Section of the National Institutes of Health in Bethesda, Maryland, which encompassed the NCI and the efforts to find compounds from plants to fight cancer. Hartwell wrote, "We have found that a sample of the 50% aqueous-ethanolic extract of the twigs of *Uncaria guianensis* showed activity in leukemia P388," but found no activity from the root extract prepared the same way.[199] Fifteen years later, Austrian researchers reported that alkaloids from the root of *Uncaria tomentosa* had shown modest activity against the same type of leukemia cells. However, they only found this activity from high concentrations of the extract—too high to be immunostimulating.[99]

Despite requests for additional root material from Brell for testing by the NCI using "new schemes,"[200,201] the results were not what the NCI had hoped for. Today, the results wouldn't be much different; the tumor-screening systems used by the NCI are not set up to test plants for immunostimulating activity.

Brell continued to work on his own. Serious interest was still being shown by scientists in Peru in 1976 when the University Cayetano purchased a supply of his extract for clinical study in patients at the Rimac Hospital in Lima.[202] After treatment with Brell's extract, 10 infants had recuperated from leukemia. Some were still in remission four years later, but the research didn't last. The year before he died, Brell wrote that the "lack of financial support, time and interest at the highest levels stopped the continuation of the studies."[152] Brell passed away in Lima, in November 1978. It seems incredible that he was only remembered for his pioneering work with cat's claw in the spring of 1995, a good 10 years after the press reported news about a medicinal vine from Peru—news that would eventually spread all over the world.[4]

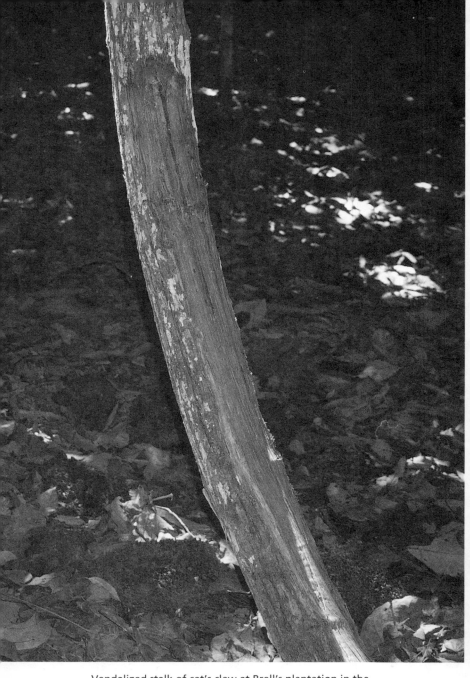

Vandalized stalk of cat's claw at Brell's plantation in the
Chanchamayo Valley, Peru

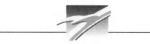

V.
Ecological Concerns

None of the local Indians in Chanchamayo, with whom I spoke, were about to dig up the root, at least not unless they were properly remunerated for their work. They explained that by leaving it to grow, the vine goes on providing a continual source of medicine, but if the root is taken, then the vine is gone. However, that isn't necessarily the case. For example, Keplinger found a way to harvest the root without disrupting the growth of the vine. He removed a portion of the main root and left the rest to grow.[10,17] Sometimes, the secondary or side-roots were taken, but only when such harvesting would not unduly compromise the continued growth of the vine.[16]

As part of quality control, the painstaking task of testing each vine for an ideal alkaloid profile before harvesting also avoids the unnecessary removal of material. But for over 10 years now, Keplinger has been cultivating cat's claw, a practice that until recently was considered the exception in Peru. Cultivars are contracted out to Asháninka Indians who raise them and are paid for their service through the purchase of the plants at the time of harvesting.[16]

The primary root grows roughly straight to highly bent and can reach several meters long, the diameter ranging in thickness from that of a finger to that of an arm. As for the secondary roots, I noticed them during my visit to Brell's old plantation. Where the vine grew half embedded along the ground, there were other side-roots as much as 10 feet away from the primary root. And where the vine came back down to the

K. Jones, 1995

ground from high up in the trees, it sent out another root before moving on and up again into the dense foliage above.

The root and stalk bark have a different appearance. The dried, coarsely ground stalk bark has a deep orange or brownish-orange color and turns to a much darker orange upon soaking or boiling in water. The dried root appears brown in color, while the wood portion in the center has an ochre color. The dried, coarsely ground root used for making tea is composed of yellowish pieces of the wood section and the reddish-brown bark portion which, under a hand lens, shows a fissured texture.[115]

In Lima I consulted a group of Peruvian forestry engineers now working with an Asháninka community in the area of Cutivireni. They informed me that initially the Indians scoffed at the idea of cultivating cat's claw, at least from seedlings. The reason seems to be their lack of familiarity with reforestation methods. But the engineers soon learned the method of planting sticks or cuttings of the vine was something the Asháninka would take seriously. Why? They suspect the reason lies in the fact the method is essentially the same one the Indians use to cultivate the main food plant in their diet, yuca (*Manihot esculenta*), which produces a starchy root. Another reason may be the Asháninka have always left the jungle to regrow by itself. The foresters I spoke with also suspect the initial ambivalence of the Asháninka to plant seedlings was due to their experience of the vine itself. After burning areas of jungle to plant their yuca, the Asháninka told them provided they hadn't removed the roots, cat's claw always came back.[203] Perhaps the banana growers on the Atlantic coast of Central America came to regard the vine as a nuisance weed[42] partly for the same reason: the vine is very persistent.

Cat's claw can also be grown from seed and there are programs underway to provide seedlings so that harvesters and future growers can plant cat's claw on a massive scale.[204,205] Guisella found a germination rate from seeds of 99.9%. However, seeds stored for a year had a germination rate of only

Ecological Concerns

30%, a problem she suspects was likely due to bacterial or fungal contamination.[206]

According to Peruvian Agricultural law (Decreed Law No. 21147), a licence must be obtained for harvesting any part of cat's claw. All parts are legal to harvest. However, as the law explains, for commercial exportation the material must be processed.[207] A tax is levied upon harvesters of cat's claw, the same as a stumpage fee for harvesting trees. But it is no more than the amount collected for the lowest grade of woods.[40]

Harvesters told me they are required to plant seedlings in the same places from which they remove any plant material, whether the root, stalk bark, or both. They also receive field instructions from forestry engineers before their harvesting licence is granted. Naturally, not everyone obtains a licence and an unknown amount of cat's claw is being extracted from the jungles by anyone who can obtain enough material to make a profit.

At least one non-governmental and non-profit organization in Peru has responded to the need of the Indians to make a decent profit from the vine without compromising their local ecology. The Association for the Conservation of the Patrimony of Cutivireni (ACPC) is a dedicated group of forestry engineers, botanists and anthropologists currently working with the Asháninka of the Ene River valley. ACPC has established programs to teach the Indians how to propagate and harvest cat's claw in ways that will insure a continued source of supply. For the stalk bark, the engineers recommend the vine be harvested at 8 inches above the ground so the stalk will grow back. They found a new stalk takes about eight years to grow from the cut vine. A mature vine is 65 to 130 feet long and, for commercial harvesting purposes, the vine must have 1.5-2 inches of inner bark. When a vine is harvested, two 8-inch sections are cut to provide one for analysis and one for planting. As mentioned earlier, the planted section, or cutting, produces roots if planted in sufficiently moist soil. Harvesting is conducted during the summer or dry season from April to September.[13]

An in-depth investigation of cat's claw by the Peruvian Institute of Rural Development was released in 1994. The Institute reported that ACPC has also instructed the Asháninka in Cutivireni in methods of processing the vine to avoid poor quality material. Noticeably infected or punctured inner bark is discarded and a drying process is made on clean, raised surfaces to avoid molding. The dried inner bark is then packaged for transport using a cotton bag packed into a plastic bag which is then placed into a polyethylene sack. Triple-bagging not only provides protection from moisture which can cause mold to grow, but also keeps out contaminants while the bark is in transport. Once the bark reaches Lima, a local university inspects and certifies each shipment.[13]

The Rural Institute report arrived at many recommendations for those who would develop cat's claw industrially. Some examples of their more critical conclusions are summarized in the following:

- The contribution of knowledge by indigenous people is "even more valuable" than scientific knowledge and deserves respect and protection through "an appropriate legislation."

- *Uncaria tomentosa* is being commercialized largely without contributing to the Indian community.

- Cat's claw must be supported with technical education at all levels, from Indian communities, to raw-material suppliers, to fabricators of cat's claw products.

- Provided adequate propagation and cultivation is implemented, the industrialization of cat's claw will contribute to the economy of the Amazon region in years to come.[13]

Vines are valued by the indigenous people of South America according to their relative abundance, strength, medicinal properties, and versatility. When a vine has a special purpose and yet occurs in limited supply, Indians are known to cultivate the species in order to insure a continual supply.[208] Their example is one for the rest of us to follow. It has been estimated that an

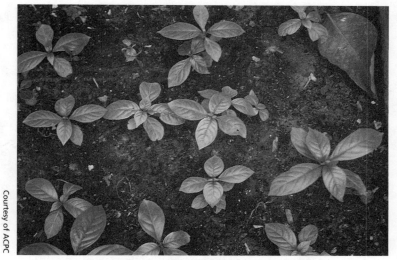

Courtesy of ACPC

Cat's claw seedlings for planting by Asháninka Indians
in Cutivireni, Peru.

indigenous culture becomes extinct with each passing year in
the Amazon basin. Since these cultures are the ones taking
most of the responsibility for protecting over 70% of the
planet's natural diversity of species,[209] plant propagation measures need to be enacted whenever and wherever high demand
for a species becomes apparent. Such measures could help preserve the lives of the very people protecting our species diversity while, at the same time, providing them with a much needed
means of legal income.

The demand for cat's claw is growing worldwide. In 1993,
Peru exported 3000 lb. of cat's claw, all to Europe. By June,
1995, exports of cat's claw expanded to include many Latin
American countries, as well as Australia and New Zealand.
Excluding the U.S., the total amount exported was over 130
tons. In 1994 the figure was one-tenth that amount.[30] In 1995
export figures for the U.S. were still not being recorded by the

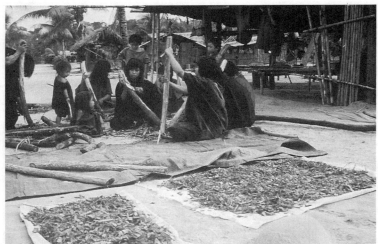

Asháninka Indians removing the inner bark of the stalk of cat's claw
for drying in Cutivireni, Peru.

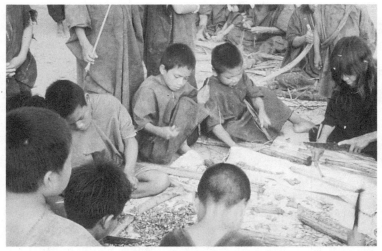

Asháninka children processing cat's claw, now the main source of income
for the tribe at Cutivireni.

Ministry of Agriculture. I estimate U.S. consumption of the stalk bark in 1994-1995 was about 200 tons.

From 1990 to 1993, the area of Iquitos exported about 2200-4400 pounds, most of it going to Lima.[210] With each vine providing 4.4 to 6.6 pounds of stalk bark,[13] that figure represents as many as 1000 vines. In 1993, cultivation of cat's claw in the area was minimal, perhaps 25-37 acres. Reforestation in the areas being harvested was practically non-existent and the locals in Iquitos continued to burn forests to plant coffee, fruits, and vegetables. Because of this, the people fear unless something is done to propagate cat's claw, it will soon vanish from central Peru.[210]

Brell recognized the problem of deforestation in 1971 and suggested a national reforestation program. He reminded the public that the very plants he had found to stimulate the immune system grew in an area of the forest that had already been "cruelly affected by the felling and burning of trees."[211] The situation was apparently well-known to the Peruvian National Institutes of Health. In a letter to Brell in 1972, they recognized that the "massive destruction of valuable botanical species is detracting from the opportunity for Peruvian scientific research to discover new plants with potential medical properties of importance."[212] Today, those same plants hold immense economic and social importance. The onus is now on the world medicinal plant industry and the government of Peru to ensure their survival.

Epilogue

A few years ago, cat's claw was almost exclusively a product of herb vendors in the streets of Peru. In the fall of 1994, cat's claw vaulted to international attention when, within one week of each other, two prominent Latin Americans told the media of the benefits they experienced from using the herb for cancer: Andreas Garcia, a TV actor with prostate cancer, and Manuel Moreyra Loredo, the highly respected former director of the Central Reserve Bank of Peru, with tumors of the brain and lung. Since their public testimonies, demand for cat's claw has skyrocketed and shows no sign of abating.[213]

A market review for the U.S. herb and vitamin industry proclaimed 1995 "the year of the cat—as in cat's claw." The sale of single herbs was up for the year from 55% in 1994 to 61% of herb sales in 1995 and cat's claw was responsible for an unknown though definitely considerable portion of the gain.[214]

On Christmas Day, 1995, *The Seattle Times* ran an article on the vine in which the Food and Drug Administration was cited, saying that as of the last week before Christmas there had been no complaints filed by anyone taking cat's claw. The article went on to report that the Government of Peru has estimated the current worth of the cat's claw industry in their country to be $100 million per year.[217] If the predictions made by some of the herb industry prophets prove accurate, cat's claw will have to be cultivated on a massive scale and immediately if Peru expects to keep up with future demand.

As I was bringing this book to a close, authorities in Russia were consulting with doctors in Peru with the idea of applying cat's claw in the treatment of people affected by the nuclear plant explosion that occurred in Chernobyl in 1987. Radioactive particles in a massive area around the plant are still causing cellular mutations in the local population—mutations that often lead to cancer. The challenge for cat's claw will be to ameliorate the ongoing damage to the immune system of those exposed to the fallout.[215]

By the end of 1995, the early efforts of Brell had been mentioned twice in the Peruvian press.[4,213] And as sensation began to give way to truth, the matter of quality finally came to the forefront. In October 1995, a consumer report on cat's claw by *El Comercio*, the leading newspaper in Peru, revealed the results of bacterial and alkaloid analyses. Of five leading encapsulated cat's claw products sold in Lima, only two were free from a pathogenic bacteria (*Pseudomonas aeruginosa*), for which the acceptable maximum allowed in such a product in Peru is zero. (*P. aeruginosa* can cause pneumonia, meningitis, and endocarditis.) Counts of aerobic bacteria in two of the products were especially high at 14,000 and 110,000—well over the maximum permitted count of 3000. And although tests showed all five products contained alkaloids (0.13% in the lowest to 0.31% in the highest), the general message of the report was buyer beware.[216]

The unprecedented market for cat's claw happened to coincide with a severe decline in the value of illicit coca crops in Peru, following the arrest of Colombian cartel members and the confiscation of significant amounts of funds which were used to purchase the crops. Peasant farmers are now beginning to seek other crops to make a living. One of the advantages of cat's claw is that it prefers supporting vegetation for shade, whereas the planting and harvesting of coca required the burning of rainforest. Unfortunately, the slow growth of cat's claw (five to 10 years before harvest) compared to coca (one to two years to become productive for five years with three to four annual harvests),[218] discourages farmers from cultivating the vine. But the opportunity is now at hand for government and industry to at least take the initiative and provide the kinds of technical support needed for alternative, and potentially lucrative, herbal crop developments in Peru. Certainly, there are other medicinal plants that could be cultivated without destroying the local ecology and with today's eager audience for herbal medicines, it only remains for them to be developed.

In response to demand and to avert the loss of woody plants such as cat's claw, the need for ecological measures with intensive nursery programs becomes more urgent, for even though the vine grows relatively fast, the root bark is "the most difficult part of a plant to obtain."[219] Thankfully, the advantages of *in vitro* culture methods for the root, already underway in Peru, offer an ecologically friendly way to produce root materials without any chance of over-harvesting wild stocks. As people around the world seek ways to avert the loss of valued species while taking advantage of their benefits, the application of this simple technology to the production of root material from other woody plants of the rainforests is expected to become more widely practiced.

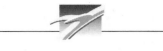

Appendix

Plants Combined with Cat's Claw
Chuchuhuasi

Chuchuhuasi (*Maytenus macrocarpa* (R. & P.) Briq.) is the bark of the trunk or root of a large extremely strong tree that grows in many parts of the Amazon. Several botanical names are given for the same tree (*M. macrocarpa=M. laevis=M. ebenifolia*).[33] The bark is unbelievably tough. I placed a two-inch piece on a sheet of 3/4-inch thick Canadian plywood and smashed it with a hammer as hard as I could. If it wasn't for the dent left in the plywood, it would be difficult to tell that the hammer had even touched the bark!

Chuchuhuasi means "trembling back," a name that may refer to its most prevalent uses.[48] The bark is commonly soaked in aguardiente rum and taken as a cure for arthritis and rheumatism, and as an aphrodisiac.[27,33] American ethnobotanist Nicole Maxwell writes that in Peru, chuchuhuasi is one of the more popular "jungle drinks" and that many of her informants insisted that for rheumatism it was the "best" remedy available.[27]

In addition to being a treatment for rheumatism and arthritis, in Peru, the bark is boiled to prepare a tea used to treat dysentery, diarrhea, upset stomach, and irregular menstrual periods.[33] In Colombia, the Siona Indians boil a small piece of the bark (5 cm) in water (2 liters) until one liter remains. To treat arthritis and rheumatism, a cup of the decoction is taken three times a day for more than a week.[34]

During the 1960s, an American pharmaceutical company

discovered that when taken orally by mice, the leaf extract produced a potent stimulating effect on the immune system, and phagocytosis was increased to a significant degree.[49] Researchers from the Catholic University in Rome, Italy, learned that the trunk bark is placed in alcohol to make a solution used to treat skin cancer. After analyzing the bark, they noted it contains high amounts of the naturally occurring antitumor substances tingenone and pristimeran, compounds classified as triterpenes.[50]

The constituents responsible for various uses of the tree in folk medicine was the subject of an article by Italian researchers at the Universita Cattolica del S. Cuore in 1982. Extracts of the trunk bark of the Colombian chuchuhuasi (*M. laevis*) had shown definite anti-inflammatory activity. Based on constituents found in the root bark, they attributed the anti-inflammatory and radiation protectant action of a water extract of the trunk bark to antioxidants, such as catechin tannins and procyanidins. They also deduced that certain triterpenes (tingenone and 22-hydroxytingenone) in chuchuhuasi, having shown antitumor activity, could account for the traditional use of the tree in treatments of skin tumors.[51]

Renewed interest in this intriguing herbal medicine appeared in 1993. Researchers at the Tokyo College of Pharmacy isolated a number of alkaloids from the tree. They note that in Peru the Indians use the "reddish-brown stem bark" soaked in rum (aguardiente) as a tonic extract taken before breakfast to treat rheumatism.[52] Perhaps in a few years we will be hearing about their success at isolating the more active constituents of this famous remedy. In the U.S., Sphinx Pharmaceutical Corporation of Durham, North Carolina, has also shown interest in chuchuhuasi. Their focus is on protein kinase C (PKC)-inhibitory components of the bark of the Ecuadorian chuchuhuasi, *Maytenus krukovii*.[53] Inhibitors of the PKC enzyme are of great interest today because there is evidence the enzyme, in an over-active state, is involved in a wide array of disease processes. Among the diseases in which PKC may be overtly involved are rheumatoid arthritis, asthma, brain tumors, cancer, and cardiovascular diseases.[54]

Chanca Piedra

The name chanca piedra means "stone-breaker" and describes one of the most common applications for this little shrub (*Phyllanthus niruri* L.): kidney stones and gallstones.[26,33] Chanca piedra is native to the tropical Americas[55] and is noted by Nicole Maxwell as one of the most promising medicinal plants she encountered in Peru. She met a doctor from Germany who had records showing that in at least 94% of cases the stones were "completely eliminated" in one or two weeks. He added that sometimes people experienced stomach cramps' which could last several hours while the stones were being expelled. Another doctor told Maxwell the herb was without side-effects and for stones it was unfailing. The German physician believed the remedy provided a "permanent" cure.[27]

During my travels in Peru, one of my guides had taken the herb for kidney stones and attested to its efficacy by claiming to be completely cured of the condition. He added that his recovery had been verified by one of the best doctors in Peru and he believed the cure to be a permanent one, too.

The real cause of kidney stones has yet to be worked out. Researchers are now focusing on calcium metabolism defects, high salt intake, and excess animal protein in the diet.[56,57] If chanca piedra proves effective for even half the annual cases of gallstones in the U.S., each year the savings would be $2.5 billion. There are, in fact, 20 million people in the U.S. who have gallstones and 600,000 cases are treated each year.[58]

In France, chanca piedra is part of a pharmaceutical preparation called Pilosuryl which is sold as a diuretic.[59] This application reflects a common use of the plant in South America. The whole plant is used in treating stones in the liver, kidney, and bladder and it is also employed to treat edema and excess uric acid. Yet, there are many other uses in the tropical Americas which merit attention. For example, the leaves and seeds are boiled with a syrup made from citrus and taken to treat jaundice or diabetes. In the Bahamas, the leaves are boiled to make a tea taken with lemon juice and salt to treat typhoid fever, flu, colds, constipation, or stomach ache. External applications are also found. In Brazil, for instance, the seeds and leaves are applied to eczema, wounds, and itches.[55]

In Peru the plant is dried and shredded to make a tea taken with lemon juice (four times a day in small doses) as a tonic for the liver. Peruvians also use the tea for pimples, inflammation of the bowels, calcifications on the ovaries, leucorrhea, stomach inflammation, diabetes, bladder or kidney stones, and ulcers.[55] The Asháninka use the plant to treat cancer, hepatitis, and diseases of the skin.[60] Peruvian chanca piedra is exported for sale in Germany. Tests by toxicologists in Germany showed chanca piedra presents no irritant or tumor-promoting actions.[55]

Brazilian researchers have gone on to find potent, "long-lasting" pain-blocking activities from the roots, stems, and leaves of various species of _Phyllanthus_.

Few efforts have been made to investigate the use of chanca piedra for treating gallstones and kidney stones. The exception was a study in Brazil by Dr. J. B. Calixto and colleagues at the Federal University of Santa Catarina in 1984. Although they used a species (_P. sellowianus_) that herbalists substitute for _P. niruri_ owing to its scarcity in the area, their results were very significant.[61] They found at least one alkaloid (phyllanthoside)[62] in the leaves and stems holds potent antispasmodic activity. The alkaloid showed potent activity as a relaxing agent for smooth muscles, especially those of the intestines. While more research was needed with preparations of the plant to confirm their findings, they concluded that the spasmolytic action could reasonably account for the use of chanca piedra in expelling stones. Calixto noted that because of this action other traditional uses of the plant might also be explained. These include the treatment of dysentery, spasmodic episodes of the intestines, and intestinal inflammation.[61]

Brazilian researchers have gone on to find potent, "long-lasting" pain-blocking activities from the roots, stems, and leaves of various species of *Phyllanthus*.[63-66] Extracts of the herbs made with alcohol and water produced pain-blocking activity in mice, whether they were injected with the extracts or received them orally. In the test system used, the extract of *Phyllanthus urinaria* showed about four times more potent activity than indomethacin and three times the strength of morphine against the second phase of pain which models the stage of "inflammatory" pain.[66] The pain model used in these tests (formalin-induced persistent pain) appears to provide a state similar to that of postoperative pain in people.[64]

One of the pain-blockers in *Phyllanthus* has been identified as gallic acid ethyl ester.[61] Other constituents, at least partly responsible for the activity, are steroidal compounds (*Beta*-sitosterol and stigmasterol).[63]

Research in Japan and India has shown the merit of chanca piedra as a liver tonic. A significant protective action was exhibited by an extract of the herb on rat liver cells subjected to cell-damaging chemicals. The primary compounds responsible were phyllanthin, hypophyllanthin and triacontanal.[67]

Two of the liver-protecting compounds have actions that may help to partly explain the use of chanca piedra by the Asháninka in the treatment of cancer. When phyllanthin and hypophyllanthin were tested for antitumor activity, there was nothing significant to report. But when they were combined with a known anticancer agent (the alkaloid vinblastine), the antitumor activity of the agent was significantly enhanced; with phyllanthin, by about four times.[68] Could it be that other alkaloids are enhanced by the presence of compounds in chanca piedra? Future research may hold the answer.

Sangre de Drago

One slash of a machete across the bark of a sangre de drago tree (*Croton lechleri* L., *C. draconoides* (Muell.) Arg. or *C. palanostigma* (Klotzschs), *C. erythrochilis*, and some other *Croton* species) and you understand the origin of its name. The blood-red sap that exudes from the cut is renowned in the Amazon for its wound-healing properties.[69] Maxwell writes that applied topically the sap stops wounds from bleeding and disinfects at the same time.[70] For these reasons sangre de drago or "dragon's blood" has been called the liquid bandage. Another common name is sangre de grado or "blood of gladness."

In Peru I had the opportunity to see this sap at work first-hand. I was visiting a friend of Nicole Maxwell's at a house on a beach near Lima. A young surfer hobbled in with a 2.5 inch cut on the inside arch of one of his feet. The cut had come from the fin of his surfboard. There was very little bleeding, no doubt due to the cold waters of the Pacific during winter on the Peruvian coast. His mother applied a few drops of the red liquid she always keeps on hand, and a small bandage was placed over the wound. I met the same surfer six hours later in the city. He was dancing as if nothing had happened and told me the cut wasn't causing him any pain. His mother reminded me that her son may have been a poor case to follow: he was as strong as a bull and built like a Viking. I suspect that many surfers in Peru use sangre de drago, for the liquid bandage is commonly known throughout the country.

Besides cuts and wounds, there are many other uses of sangre de drago in the region of the Amazon that are equally, if not more, fascinating. In Ecuador, the Quijos Quichua people treat hives by drinking the sap (20 drops) mixed with pineapple juice (200 ml). They also take the sap internally to cure diar-

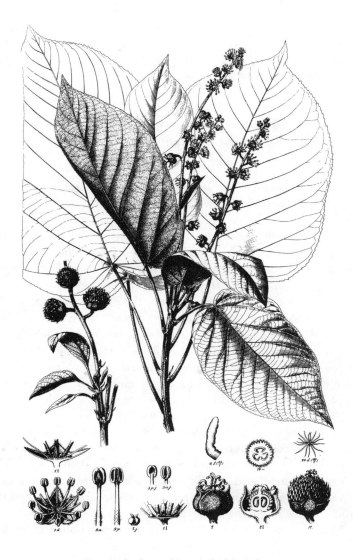

Sangre de drago (*Croton lechleri* L.).

From Carlos F. P. De Martius and Augustus G. Eichler, Flora Brasiliensis, 1873-1874, vol. 2, part 2. (Weinheim, Germany: Verlag von J. Cramer, 1967), reprint.

rhea, apply it in the mouth to treat infected gums, and for relief from the pain of cavities and tooth extractions.[48] Around Manaus, Brazil, the sap is a common folk remedy used topically to relieve the pain of boils and ulcers.[34]

In the Peruvian Amazon, sangre de drago is very often used to treat diarrhea and flu.

In northwestern Peru, shamans prescribe the sap for external use to heal wounds and for internal use as a tonic, an antidote for poisoning, and as an antitumor medicine.[31] Native peoples in the region of Pucallpa, Peru have also used the sap for the treatment of tumors[71] and this use can still be found among the Asháninka. Their name for the tree is "irare."[60] In Peru the sap is also used in treating rheumatism,[72] hemorrhoids, leucorrhea, fractures, and in the recovery from dangerous burns.[26] In the Peruvian Amazon, sangre de drago is very often used to treat diarrhea and flu. Other internal uses in this region include tonsillitis, tuberculosis, intestinal disorders, herpes, fertility-enhancement,[73] stomach ulcers,[33] and the stanching of excessive bleeding of the vagina following childbirth.[73] In the latter application, the sap is diluted in water to make a wash.[74]

Extensive surveys of traditional uses of the sap show that the most common internal applications are for stomach ulcers, lung problems, diarrhea, coughs, and flu. The usual dosage is five to ten drops diluted in alcohol, milk, or water, taken one to three times daily for five days. Externally applied, the most common uses for the sap are in healing cuts, herpes, open sores, and the gums following tooth extractions.[74]

The amount of scientific research already applied to understanding sangre de drago is immense. Patents have been issued for its use as an antiviral agent,[73] a wound-healing agent,[75] and an anti-inflammatory preparation.[76] In addition, the traditional use of the sap to treat tumors appears to have some basis.

An alkaloid in the sap called taspine inhibited viruses known to cause cancers, such as sarcoma (simian sarcoma virus type I) and leukemia (Rauscher murine leukemia virus). The action of taspine on these viruses was directed at an enzyme called reverse transcriptase, which certain viruses use to replicate in normal cells. Inhibitors of this enzyme system may therefore inhibit the development of certain cancers in man.[77] Taspine has also shown strong activity against tumor cells in cultures.[78] Tested for tumor-*promoting* activity or a carcinogenic action in mice, taspine showed no activity after 17 months. The sap was also devoid of carcinogenic activity.[79]

The sap contains an incredible amount of compounds known as proanthocyanidins, or condensed tannins.[74] By dry weight, they make up as much as 90% of the sap and are soluble. This group of plant chemicals is largely composed of tannins of a type known as catechins.[80] In the treatment of cuts, wounds, burns, and other tissue injuries, these compounds bind to and precipitate proteins and form a crust at the injury site, an action that helps to protect the skin while it heals.[81]

A press release on October 16, 1995, by Shaman Pharmaceuticals, Inc. of South San Francisco, California, reported that proanthocyanidins extracted from sangre de drago are useful in the treatment of *Herpes simplex* and watery diarrhea, which is caused by bacterial infections such as cholera and *E. coli*. With 26 million prescriptions for infectious diarrheal diseases annually, Shaman Pharmaceuticals could play a major role in countering one of the world's most prevalent diseases. And, as many travelers are aware, severe dehydration from infectious diarrhea can be fatal.

Herpes simplex is much more prevalent than generally recognized. With at least 50% of adults worldwide now showing positive in tests to detect exposure to the virus, the need for effective treatments is long overdue.

Shaman has isolated particular proanthocyanidins from the sap,[73] which are now undergoing the necessary lengthy tests in people. They have been testing a large water-soluble proanthocyanidin compound called SP-303. Described as an oligomeric composed of a number of condensed catechin tannins, SP-303 is a dark red-brown powder that turns light brown and fluffy when freeze-dried. Applied in the form of an ointment, SP-303 has shown good activity against genital herpes (HSV-2) in guinea pigs and mice. SP-303 is currently undergoing clinical trials[74] in people with genital herpes and in others with secretory diarrhea. If the results are as good as those found in their laboratory, sangre de drago may be something everyone will be hearing about on the six-o'clock news.

Dr. Pieters found that the raw sangre de drago sap had caused a superior healing.

As part of sangre de drago's wound-healing effects, a significant anti-inflammatory action is attributed to the alkaloid taspine. In rats that received taspine hydrochloride orally, there was three to four times more anti-inflammatory activity than that of phenylbutazone in the same doses. In tests for antiarthritic activity, the alkaloid also produced significant results when taken orally and at doses well below what could be toxic.[72] Consequently, various formulations of taspine hydrochloride have been proposed for use in treating inflammatory conditions. These include ointments, tablets, capsules, powders, and lozenges.[76]

The primary wound-healing element of the sap has been determined by some to be the alkaloid taspine[73,80] and by others as something entirely different: a lignan (3',-0-dimethylcedrusin) which I'll call DMC for short.[69,81,82] The lignan has shown a definite protective effect against the break-down of cells and it was effective in the lab in the same general amounts in which it occurs in the sap.[82]

But what do scientists really know about the wound-healing action of the sap itself?

Experiments at the Universidad Peruano Cayetano Heredia in Lima, Peru, showed that even the diluted sap as 10% of a topical solution increased the healing rate of wounds to a significant degree. Compared to mice not treated with the solution, after five applications in two days the wounds responded to sangre de drago so well they showed a 31% greater completion of healing.[80]

Similar studies were conducted by Dr. Luc Pieters at the University of Antwerp in Belgium, a country where the sap is already being sold in pharmacies. Applying the raw, undiluted sap, Dr. Pieters found that wound tissue was already contracted after 24 hours and the whole area of the wounds had developed a protective dark crust. It was under the microscope that the full impact of the remarkable healing sap could be more fully appreciated; there was practically no difference between the new tissue that had just formed and the old skin that had not been disturbed. In fact, the entire formation of the new layer of skin was nearly complete.[69]

Comparing the results produced from the same test procedure using the alkaloid taspine, or compared to wounds left to heal by themselves, Dr. Pieters found the raw sangre de drago sap produced a superior healing. There were even newly formed hair follicles. When he compared the effects to those of an ointment containing the lignan DMC (0.05%), there were more hair follicles and a more developed layer of outer skin from application of the crude sap. Even though Dr. Pieters identified the lignan as "the biologically active" wound-healing principle in the sap, it was clear the old remedy worked best, just the way it was. And this, he learned, was because of the excellent crust-forming action of the catechin tannins abundant in the sap.[69]

In the treatment of cancer, sangre de drago appears to lend support to the healing of tissues but doesn't appear to be an anticancer substance by itself. It also provides a certain antibiotic effect against various harmful bacteria (*Bacillus subtilis* and *Escherichia coli*). As nature would have it, the levels of taspine in the trees show great variation from one area to the next. It has therefore been suggested when taspine levels are low the sap may be acting more as an immune system stimulant than as any directly tumor-cell-destroying agent. When the levels are higher, traditional use of the sap as an antitumor agent may be more direct. Some researchers now conclude that taken together, these actions may well account for sangre de drago's traditional use as a tumor remedy in Peru.[83]

The sap cannot be easily tapped like the latex of rubber trees, but the rapid growth and wide range of sangre de drago trees, coupled with high yields of the sap from scoring the bark of fallen trees (1.3-1.5 gallons/tree), or from standing trees (several quarts),[74] means there is little likelihood of extinction.

Like "uña de gato," chuchuhuasi and sangre de drago are common names given to other plants besides the ones discussed here. For that reason it is imperative to obtain medicinal plant products from reliable sources who have taken the steps necessary to assure authentic material. Quality standards associations and professional organizations of herbalists in your area can direct you to companies that supply products in compliance with the required criteria.

A Look at the Leaves

The activity of the leaves of *U. tomentosa* had shown a "slightly higher" rate of immune potentiation than the stalk bark, even though the batch tested held *no* isopteropodine. Yet the leaves of another harvest two years earlier did contain the alkaloid. When the alkaloids were in amounts comparable to those of the root, the leaves produced increases in immune system activity of "between 30% and 40%"—the same as the root.[100]

Actions of Alkaloids in the Leaves and Stems (*Uncaria tomentosa* and *U. guianensis*)[106]

Hirsutine

Inhibits urinary bladder contractions[107]
Inhibits gastric erosions[108]
Blood vessel-relaxing[109]
Mild antispasmodic[110]
Local anesthetic[111]
Anti-arrhythmic[108]

Rynchophylline

Causes peripheral blood vessels to dilate
Temporarily lowers blood pressure
Lowers blood cholesterol
Stimulates respiration[112]
Mild antispasmodic[110]
(Also in stalk bark and root[95])

Isorynchophylline

Immunostimulating[99]
Mild antispasmodic[110]
(Also in stalk bark and root[95])

Dihydrocorynantheine

Potentially active against headaches
(5-hydroxytryptamine antagonist)[113]
Mild antispasmodic[110]

Upon learning this, I was immediately reminded of the Indians in Suriname who used the dried and powdered leaves of cat's claw (*U. guianensis*) to treat wounds.[35,36] And while the Cashibo rolled the leaves into little poultices to cure abscesses,[13] it was the Asháninka who used the tea of the boiled bark for the purpose of treating wounds.[43] Since wound-healing is part of the many tasks the immune system performs to keep us well,[104] an accelerated healing of wounds might well be expected from an immune potentiator. It came as little surprise, then, to find that in Europe doctors had already anticipated an ointment containing the alkaloids of cat's claw.[100] However, my curiosity about the leaves persisted.

At the School of Pharmacy in London, England, in 1974, Drs. S. R. Hemingway and J. D. Phillipson found that in the leaves of both species of cat's claw, the main oxindole alkaloids were isorynchophylline and rynchophylline. In addition, they found other kinds of alkaloids in the leaves, such as hirsutine and dihydrocorynantheine (heteroyohimbine alkaloids).[106] Each of these alkaloids has been the subject of activity studies that may help to explain certain folk-uses of the leaves.

Variable Levels of Alkaloids

As you can see from the following chart, even in one color variety of cat's claw there are considerable variations in levels of immunologically-active alkaloids from one year to another.

Uncaria tomentosa (Root Bark)
Yellow-Brown Variety

Dates	10/1985	06/1983	08/1981
Isopteropodine	0.15	0.01	0.16
Pteropodine	0.48	0.04	0.48
Mitraphylline	1.04	0.04	0.76
Isomitraphylline	0.38	0.05	0.26
Isorynchophylline	7.17	0.12	8.86
Speciophylline	0.35	0.02	0.28
Totals (mg/gram)	9.57	0.28	10.8

Adapted from Laus, G. and D. Keplinger.[101]

Safety Concerns

After all the positive findings regarding cat's claw, the reader may well ask if something as simple as an herbal tea or extract can improve the odds of patients surviving, why hasn't it become more widely used? The simple answer is that the wheel of medicine grinds exceedingly slow. No matter how long a substance has been in use in folk medicine, it still requires clinical testing before most physicians will even consider it. This kind of testing usually takes cooperative funding and years of time. Thankfully, for those who are sick or facing death and don't have time to wait, the root and the bark of cat's claw are not toxic.[100,139]

I found no indications in the literature that *Uncaria tomentosa* or *U. guianensis* taken in traditional dosages are in any way toxic. In mice, the water extract of the root bark (*U. tomentosa*) taken orally produced no toxicity in a dosage of five grams per kilogram of body weight.[100]

According to Brell, the best way to prepare cat's claw was to make a 50% alcohol/water tincture by letting the root bark soak rather than boiling it.[155] Because the pentacyclic alkaloids in cat's claw are only slightly water-soluble but easily dissolve in alcohol (and dilute acids), Brell's method offered an efficient preparation.

As an extra precaution until more is known, cat's claw in any form should be avoided by pregnant women, those planning to become pregnant, and by anyone breast-feeding. Also, anyone who has recently had, or is planning, skin grafts or organ transplants must not take cat's claw, or any other immunostimulant, at least not until their system has returned to normal. A person doing so runs the risk of their immune system rejecting the newly transplanted cells.[7]

As previously noted, children under the age of three are forbidden to take the root in any form in Austria. Several other precautions are given in Europe for proprietary products of cat's claw. Although they specifically pertain to the use of standardized, pentacyclic oxindole alkaloid-rich products used by physicians,[7] the precautions may also apply to other cat's claw products. Indeed, they may also apply to other kinds of immunostimulants, herbal or otherwise.

When hemophiliacs are receiving therapy with cryoprecipitates or fresh blood plasma, the prescription cat's claw products available in Austria and Germany are avoided in any "concurrent administration." However, taken at the same time as standardized blood plasma factor for hemophiliacs hasn't presented a problem. Physicians are also warned not to combine cat's claw with passive vaccines composed of animal sera, nor with intravenous hyperimmunoglobulin therapy, intravenous thymic extracts, insulin (bovine or porcine in origin), or other hormone therapies "with animal proteo or peptide hormones."[7] If you have any doubts about combining cat's claw with other products you may be taking, it would be prudent to check with your doctor first.

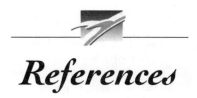

References

1. "Darían a la 'uña de gato' estatus oficial de planta medicinal," *El Comercio* (Lima), April 9, 1994.

2. "Uña de Gato" será Mundialmente Reconocida como Medicina en Ginebra: Campas y Asháninkas beben Infusión de Liana para Curar Determinados Males," *Diario La Republica*, April 12, 1994: 12.

3. Cabieses, Fernando, *The Saga of Cat's Claw* (Lima, Peru: Via Lactea Editores, 1994).

4. Hidalgo, José Luis, "Historia de un Escamoteo," *El Mundo* (Lima), April 22-23, 1995: E3.

5. Whitworth, Eugene, personal communication, June 8 and July 2, 1995.

6. *Krallendorn®-Drugs: A Brief Survey* (Volders, Austria: Immodal Pharmaka, September 1994), brochure.

7. *Krallendorn,® Uncaria tomentosa (Willd.) DC Root Extract: Information for Physicians and Dispensing Chemists*, 3rd revised edition (Volders, Austria: Immodal Pharmaka GmbH, September 1995), 20 pp.

8. Miró-Quesada Cantuarias, Oscar, Institutos Nacionales de Salud, Lima, letter to Arturo Brell, November 23, 1970.

9. "Gibt es wirksame Heilpflanze gegen Krebs?" *Der Algauer* no. 203, September 3, 1965.

10. Keplinger, Deitmar, Volders, Austria, personal communication, October 4, 1995.

11. Schatz, Wilfried, "Ashaninka-kind Sally besuchte großzügige Stanzer Schulkinder," *Tiroler Tageszeitung*, March 19, 1993: 31.

12. Bartle, Jim, *Parque Nacional Huascaran Ancas, Peru* (Lima, Peru: Asociacion Peruana Para la Conservación de la Naturaleza, 1985).

13. Ocampo T., Palmiro, ed., *Uncaria tomentosa, Aspectos Etnomédicos, Médicos, Farmacológicos, Botánicos, Agrónomicos, Comerciales, Legales, Antropológicos, Sociales y Políticos* (Lima, Peru: Instituto de Desarrollo Rural Peruano (IDDERP), 1994), 74 pp.

14. Schuler S., Luis, Gerónimo Schuler Egg, Martha Schuler Egg, and Herminio Schuler Egg, letter to Arturo Brell, August 10, 1974.

15. Nadramia, Maria Christina, "La Uña de Gato Cura el Cancer," *Gente* (Lima), August 29, 1974: 8-9.

16. Keplinger, Ursula, personal communication, November 6, 1995.

17. Keplinger, Klaus, personal communication, November 7, 1995.

18. Egg, Augustín Schuler, "Investigación y Trabajos de Campo Sobre lo uña de gato en Pozuzo," *Despertar Pozucino* no. 5, July 1995: 53-54.

19. Keplinger, K., "Composition Allowing for Modifying the Growth of Living Cells, Preparation and Utilization of Such a Composition," Internationale Veroffentlichungsdatum WO 82/01130, April 15, 1982.

20. Steward, J. H., "Tribes of the Montana and Bolivian Andes," Julian H. Steward, ed., *Handbook of South American Indians*, 3 (Smithsonian Institution Bureau of American Ethnology: Washington, DC, 1948): 507-533.

21. Keplinger, Klaus, *Der Baum, der einem Mann ein Kind Schenkte: Indianische Märchen und Mythen aus dem Regenwald* (Frieburg, Germany: Herder/Spektrum, 1993).

22. "Tiroler enträtselt Indianerschrift," *Der Standard*, July 3/4, 1993: 25.

23. Keplinger, Klaus, Das Shevátari: Eine Vergessene Schrift aus dem peruanischen Urwald (Innsbruck, Austria: Österreichischer Studenien Verlag, 1993).

24. Plotkin, Mark J., *Tales of a Shaman's Apprentice* (New York, NY: Penguin Books, 1993): 104-105.

25. Steward, Julian H. and Alfred Métraux, "Tribes of the Peruvian and Ecuadorian Montana" in Julian H. Steward (ed.), *Handbook of South American Indians* 3 (Washington, DC: U.S. Government Printing Office, 1948): 535-649.

26. Rutter, Richard A., *Catologo de Plantas Utiles de la Amazonia Peruana* (Pucallpa, Peru: Ministerio de Educacion, Instituto Lingüístico de Verano, 1990).

27. Maxwell, Nicole, *Witch Doctor's Apprentice* (New York, NY: Citadel Press, 1990): 363-381.

28. Maxwell, Nicole, "Jungle Pharmacy," *South American Explorer* 1, no. 4 (1979): 8-13.

29. Vilches, Lida E. Obregon, *Uña De Gato* (Lima, Peru: Instituto de Fitoterapia Americano, 1994), in Spanish.

30. Carrillo, Cesar Adolfo Zavala, *Taxonomía, distribución eco-geográfica y status del Género Uncaria Schreb. (Uña de gato), en el Peru*, Thesis, Universidad Nacional Agraria La Molina, Lima, Peru, 1995.

31. De Feo, V., "Medicinal and Magical Plants in the Northern Peruvian Andes," *Fitoterapia* 63 (1992): 417-440.

32. Tanaka, Tyozaburo, *Tanaka's Cyclopedia of Edible Plants of the World*, Sasuke Nakao, ed. (Tokyo: Keigaku Publishing Co., 1976): 746-747.

33. Duke, James A. and Rodolfo Vasquez, *Amazonian Ethnobotanical Dictionary* (Boca Raton, Fl: CRC Press, 1994).

34. Schultes, Richard Evans and Robert E. Raffauf, *The Healing Forest, Medicinal and Toxic Plants of the Northwest Amazonia* (Portland, Or: Dioscorides Press, 1990).

35. Ostendorf, F. W., "Nuttige Planten en Sierplanten in Suriname," *Landbouwproefstation Suriname Bulletin* no. 79 (1962): 199-200.

36. Raymond-Hamet, M., "Sur l'Alcaloide Principal d'une Rubiaceé des Régions Tropicales de l'Amérique de Sud: *l'Ourouparia guianensis* Aubelt," *Comptes Rendus Hebdomadaires des Séances de L'Académie des Sciences* 235 (1952): 547-550.

37. Yépez, A. M. et al., "Quinovic Acid Glycosides from *Uncaria guianensis*," *Phytochemistry* 30 (1991): 1635-1637.

38. Ridsdale, C. E., "A Revision of *Mitragyna* and *Uncaria* (Rubiacea)," *Blumea* 24 (1978): 43-100.

39. Standley, P. C., "The Rubiaceae of Venezuela," *Field Museum of Natural History, Botanical Series* 7, no. 4 (1931): 354.

40. Brell, Guisella Tesoro, personal communication, August 7 and October 25, 1995.

41. Woodson, R. E. and R. W. Schery, "Flora of Panama Part IX Family 179. Rubiaceae—Part II, John D. Dwyer," *Annals of the Missouri Botanical Garden* 67 (1980): 257-522.

42. Standley, P. C., "Flora of Costa Rica," *Field Museum of Natural History, Botanical Series* 18, part 4 (1930): 1379.

43. "Uña de Gato Asháninka," ACPC (Lima, Peru: Association for the Conservation of the Patrimony of Cutivireni), 4 pp., undated.

44. Medina, Javier Aroca and Luis Maury Parra, "El Pueblo Asháninka de la Selva Central: Estado, Derecho y Pueblos Indígenas," *America Indigena* 53, no. 4 (1993): 11-32.

45. Gorriti, G., "Terror in the Andes: The Flight of the Ashaninkas," *The New York Times Magazine*, Dec. 2, 1990: 40-44,48,65-66,68, and 71-72. See also, Gagnon, Friar Mariano, *Warriors in Eden* (New York, NY: William Morrow and Company, 1993).

46. Miranda, Hector J. Vega (ACPC), Lima, letter to the author, September 1, 1995.

47. *Manejemos Nuestra Uña de Gato: Uncaria tomentosa, Uncaria guianensis* (Lima, Peru: Association for the Conservation of the Patrimony of Cutivireni), 16 pp., undated.

48. Marles, R. J., *The Ethnopharmacology of the Lowland Quichua of Eastern Ecuador*, dissertation of the University of Illinois at Chicago, 1988 (Ann Arbor, MI: University Microfilms International, 1992).

49. DiCarlo, F. J. et al., "Reticuloendothelial System Stimulants of Botanical Origin," *Journal of the Reticuloendothelial Society* 1 (1964): 224-232.

50. Martinod, P. et al., "Isolation of Tingenone and Pristimerin from *Maytenus chuchuhuasca*," *Phytochemistry* 15 (1976): 562-563.

51. Gonzalez Gonzalez, J. et al., "Chuchuhuasha—A Drug Used in Folk Medicine in the Amazonian and Andean Areas. A Chemical Study of *Maytenus laevis*," *Journal of Ethnopharmacology* 5 (1982): 73-77.

52. Itokawa, H. et al., "Oligo-Nicotinated Sesquiterpene Polyesters from *Maytenus ilicifolia*," *Journal of Natural Products* 56 (1993): 1479-1485.

53. Sekar, Kumara V. S. et al., "Mayteine and 6-Benzoyl-6-deacetyl-mayteine from *Maytenus krukovii*," *Planta Medica* 61 (1995): 390.

54. Bradshaw, D. et al., Therapeutic Potential of Protein Kinase C Inhibitors," *Agents and Actions* 38 (1993): 135-147.

55. Unander, D. W. et al., "Uses and Bioassays in *Phyllanthus* (Euphorbiaceae): A Compilation II. The Subgenus *Phyllanthus*," *Journal of Ethnopharmacology* 34 (1991): 97-133.

56. Martinez-Maldonado, Manuel, "How to Avoid Kidney Stones," *The Saturday Evening Post*, September/October 1995: 36-38.

57. SerVaas, Cory et al., "If You Have a Kidney Stone, Know What Kind," *The Saturday Evening Post*, September/October 1995: 40, 41, 88

58. "NIH Consensus Conference: Gallstones and Laparoscopic Cholecystectomy," *Journal of the American Medical Association* 269 (February 24, 1993): 1018-1024.

59. Weninger, Bernard and Lionel Robineau, *Elements for a Caribbean Pharmacopeia* (Dominican Republic: Enda-Caribe, 1988): 202-204.

60. Reynel, Carlos et al., *Etnobotanica Campa-Ashaninca, Con Especial Referencias las Especies del Bosque Secundario* (Lima, Peru: Facultad de Ciencias Forestales de la Universidad Nacional Agraria La Molina, 1990).

61. Calixto, J. B. et al., "Antispasmodic Effects of an Alkaloid Extracted from *Phyllanthus sellowianus*: A Comparative Study with Papaverine," *Brazilian Journal of Biological Research* 17 (1984): 313-321.

62. Miguel, G. et al., "A Triterpene and Phenolic Compounds from Leaves and Stems of *Phyllanthus sellowianus*," *Planta Medica* 61 (1995): 391.

63. Santos, A. R. S. et al., "Antinociceptive Properties of Steroids Isolated from *Phyllanthus corcovadensis* in Mice," *Planta Medica* 61 (1995): 329-332.

64. Gorski, F. et al., "Potent Antinociceptive Activity of a Hydroalcoholic Extract of *Phyllanthus corcovadensis*," *Journal of Pharmacy and Pharmacology* 45 (1993): 1046-1049.

65. Santos, A. R. S. et al., "Analgesic Effects of Callus Culture Extracts from Selected Species of *Phyllanthus* in Mice," *Journal of Pharmacy and Pharmacology* 46 (1994): 755-759.

66. Santos, A. R. S. et al., "Further Studies on the Antinociceptive Action of the Hydroalcoholic Extracts from Plants of the Genus *Phyllanthus*," *Journal of Pharmacy and Pharmacology* 47 (1995): 66-71.

67. Syamasundar, K. V. et al., "Antihepatotoxic Principles of *Phyllanthus niruri*," *Journal of Ethnopharmacology* 14 (1985): 41-44.

68. Somanabandhu, A. et al., "^{1}H- and ^{13}C-NMR Assignments of Phyllanthin and Hypophyllanthin: Lignans that Enhance Cytotoxic Responses with Cultured Multidrug-Resistant Cells," *Journal of Natural Products* 56 (1993): 233-239.

69. Pieters, Luc, *The Biologically Active Constituents of "Sangre de Drago," a Traditional South American Drug*, dissertation of the Department of Farmaceutische Wetenschappen of the University of Antwerp, Belgium, 1992 (Ann Arbor, MI: University Microfilms International, 1995).

70. Maxwell, Nicole, *Witch Doctor's Apprentice* (New York, NY: Citadel Press, 1990): 293.

71. Hartwell, J. L., "Plants Used Against Cancer: A Survey," *Lloydia* 32 (1969): 158-176.

72. Perdue, G. P. et al., "South American Plants II: Taspine Isolation and Anti-Inflammatory Activity," *Journal of Pharmaceutical Sciences* 68 (1979): 124-126.

73. Tempesta, M. S., "Proanthocyanidin Polymers having Antiviral Activity and Methods of Obtaining Same," United States Patent 5,211,944, May 18, 1993.

74. Ubillas, R. et al., "SP-303, an Antiviral Oligomeric Proanthocyanidin from the Latex of *Croton lechleri* (Sangre de Drago)," *Phytomedicine* 1 (1994): 77-106. See also, David Riggle, "Pharmaceuticals from the Rainforest," *In Business*, January/February, 1992: 26-29.

75. Lewis, W. H. et al., "Wound-Healing Composition," United States Patent 5,156,847, October 20, 1992.

76. Persinos, G. J., "Anti-inflammation Compositions Containing Taspine or Acid Salts Thereof and Method of Use," United States Patent 3,694,557, September 26, 1972.

77. Sethi, M. L., "Inhibition of RNA-Directed DNA Polymerase Activity of RNA Tumor Viruses by Taspine," *Canadian Journal of Pharmaceutical Sciences* 12 (1977): 7-9.

78. Itokawa, H. et al., "A Cytotoxic Substance from Sangre de Grado," *Chemical and Pharmaceutical Bulletin* 39 (1991): 1041-1042.

79. Vaisberg, A. J. et al., "Taspine is the Cicatrizant Principle in Sangre de Grado Extracted from *Croton lechleri*," *Planta Medica* 55 (1989): 140-143.

80. Cai, Y. et al., "Polyphenolic Compounds from *Croton lechleri*," *Phytochemistry* 30 (1991): 2033-2040.

81. Pieters, L. et al., "*In Vitro* and *In Vivo* Biological Activity of South American Dragon's Blood and its Constituents," *Planta Medica* 58, suppl. 1 (1992): A582-A583.

82. Pieters, L. et al., "Isolation of a Dihydrobenzofuran Lignan from South American Dragon's Blood (*Croton* Spp.) as an Inhibitor of Cell Proliferation," *Journal of Natural Products* 56 (1993): 899-906.

83. Chen, Z.-P. et al., "Studies on the Antitumor, Anti-bacterial, and Wound-Healing Properties of Dragon's Blood," *Planta Medica* 60 (1994): 541-545.

84. "Control de fábricas procesadoras de 'uña de gato' debe ser estricto," *El Comercio* (Lima), Tuesday, October 17, 1995.

85. Davis, E. Wade, "Ethnobotany: An Old Practice, A New Discipline," in R. E. Schultes and Siri von Reis (eds.), *Ethnobotany: Evolution of a Discipline* (Portland, OR: Dioscorides Press, 1995): 40-51.

86. Morell, Virginia, "Jungle Prescriptions," *International Wildlife*, May/June, 1984: 18-24.

87. Bisset, Norman G., "Arrow Poisons and Their Role in the Development of Medicinal Agents," R. E. Schultes and Siri von Reis (eds.), *Ethnobotany: Evolution of a Discipline* (Portland, OR: Dioscorides Press, 1995): 289-302.

88. Senatore, A. et al., "Ricerche Fitochimiche e Biologiche Sull *Uncaria tomentosa*," *Bollettino Societa di Biologia Sperimentale* 65 (1989): 517-520.

89. Fazzi, Marco A. Costa, *Evaluation de la Uncaria tomentosa (Uña de Gato) en lan Prevencion de Ulceras Gastricas de Stress Producidas Experimentalmente en Rats* (Dissertation of the Faculty of Medicine, University Peruana Cayetano Heredia, Lima, Peru, 1989).

90. Cerri, R. et al., "New Quinovic Acid Glycosides from *Uncaria tomentosa*," *Journal of Natural Products* 51 (1988): 257-261.

91. Aquino, R. et al., "Plant Metabolites. New Compounds and Anti-Inflammatory Activity of *Uncaria tomentosa*," *Journal of Natural Products* 54 (1991): 453-459.

92. Yasukawa, K. et al., "Effect of Chemical Constituents from Plants on 12-*O*-Tetradecanoylphorbol-13-acetate-Induced Inflammation in Mice," *Chemical and Pharmaceutical Bulletin* 37 (1989): 1071-1073.

93. Recio, M. C. et al., "Structural Requirements for the Anti-Inflammatory Activity of Natural Triterpenoids," *Planta Medica* 61, no. 2 (1995): 182-185.

94. Arroyo, J. et al., "Avances en la Evaluación Farmacológica de los Extractos de *Uncaria guianensis*," in *II Congreso Italo-Peruano de Etnomedicina Andina*, Lima, Peru, October 27-30, 1993 (Lima, Peru: Sociedad Italo-Andina de Etnomedicina): 24-25.

95. Kreutzkamp, Barbara, *Niedermolekulare Inhalstoffe mit Immunstimulierenden Eigenschaften aus Uncaria tomentosa, Okoubaka aubrevillei und anderen Drogen* (Dissertation of the Faculty of Chemistry and Pharmacy of Ludwig Maximilians University, Munich, May 1984).

96. Lewis, W. H. and M. P. F. Elvin-Lewis, *Medical Botany: Plants Affecting Man's Health* (New York, NY: John Wiley and Sons, 1977).

97. Stuppner, H. et al., "HPLC Analysis of the Main Oxindole Alkaloids from *Uncaria tomentosa*," *Chromatographia* 34, no. 11/12 (1992): 597-600.

98. Jones, Kenneth, *Pau d'Arco, Immune Power from the Rain Forest* (Rochester, VT: Healing Arts Press, 1995), *Shiitake, The Healing Mushroom* (Rochester, VT: Healing Arts Press, 1995), and *Reishi, Ancient Herb for Modern Times* by Kenneth Jones (Seattle, WA: Sylvan Press, 1992).

99. Wagner, H. et al., "Die Alkaloide von *Uncaria tomentosa* und ihre Phagozytose-steigernde Wirkung," *Planta Medica* 51 (1985): 419-423.

100. Keplinger, H., "Oxindole Alkaloids Having Properties Stimulating the Immunologic System and Preparation Containing Same," United States Patent 5,302,611, April 12, 1994.

101. Laus, G. and D. Keplinger, "Separation of Sterioisomeric Oxindole Alkaloids from *Uncaria tomentosa* by High Performance Liquid Chromatography," *Journal of Chromatography A* 662 (1994): 243-249.

102. Stuppner, Hermann, University of Innsbruck, Austria, Institute of Pharmacognosy, letter to the author, May 12, 1994.

103. Lavault, M. et al., "Alcaloides de L'*Uncaria guianensis*," *Planta Medica* 47 (1983): 244-245.

104. Cácerea, N. C., "Contribución al Químico de una especie de *Uncaria* II," *Revista de Química* 9 (1995): 66.

105. Staquet, M.-J. et al., "Expression of ICAM-3 on Human Epidermal Dendritic Cells," *Immunobiology* 192 (1995): 249-261.

106. Hemingway, S. R. and J. D. Phillipson, "Alkaloids from S. American Species of *Uncaria* (Rubiaceae)," *Journal of Pharmacy and Pharmacology* 26, suppl. (1974): 113P.

107. Ozaki, Y. and M. Harada, "Site of the Ganglion Blocking Action of Gardneramine and Hirsutine in the Dog Urinary Bladder in Situ Preparation," *Japanese Journal of Pharmacology* 33 (1983): 463-471.

108. Ozaki, Y. et al., "Pharmacological Studies on *Uncaria* and *Amsonia* Alkaloids," *Japanese Journal of Pharmacology* (suppl.) 30 (1980): 137P.

109. Yano, S. et al., "Ca^{2+} Channel Blocking Effects of Hirsutine, an Indole Alkaloid from *Uncaria* Genus, in the Isolated Rat Aorta," *Planta Medica* 57 (1991): 403-405.

110. Ozaki, Y., "Pharmacological Studies of Indole Alkaloids Obtained from Domestic Plants, *Uncaria rynchophylla* Miq. and *Amsonia elliptica* Roem et Schult," *Nippon Yakurigaku Zasshi* no. 1 (1994): 17-26.

111. Harada, M. et al., "Effects of Indole Alkaloids from *Gardneria nutans* Sieb. et Zucc, and *Uncaria rynchophylla* Miq. on a Guinea Pig Urinary Bladder Preparation in Situ," *Chemical and Pharmaceutical Bulletin* 27 (1979): 1069-1074.

112. Kuramochi, T. et al., "Gou-teng (from *Uncaria rynchophylla* Miquel)-induced Endothelium-dependent and -independent Relaxations in the Isolated Rat Aorta," *Life Sciences* 54 (1994): 2061-2069.

113. Kanatani, H. et al., "The Active Principles of the Branchlet and Hook of *Uncaria sinensis* Oliv. Examined with a 5-hydroxytryptamine Receptor Binding Assay," *Journal of Pharmacy and Pharmacology* 37 (1985): 401-404.

114. Tizard, Ian R., *Immunology: An Introduction* (New York, NY: Saunders College Publishing, 1984): 52-54.

115. *Der Krallendorn® Tee* (Innsbruck, Austria: Immodal Pharmaka), 24 pp., undated clinical brochure.

116. Montenegro De Matta, S. et al., "Alkaloids and Procyanidins of an *Uncaria* sp. from Peru," *Il Farmaco Ed. Sc.* 31 (1976): 527-535.

117. Keplinger, Ursula, letter to the author, December 20, 1995.

118. "Wunder-Wurzel" aus dem Urwald heilte Gehirntumor" *Quick* magazine, 47 (1986).

119. Moss, Ralph W., *Questioning Chemotherapy* (Brooklyn, NY: Equinox Press, 1995).

120. Stuppner, H. et al., "A Differential Sensitivity of Oxindole Alkaloids to Normal and Leukemic Cell Lines," *Planta Medica* 59, suppl. (1993): A583.

121. Peluso, G. et al., "Effetto Antiproliferativo su Cellule Tumorali di Estrattie Metaboliti da *Uncaria tomentosa*. Studi in vitro Sulla Loro Azione DNA Polimerasi," II Congreso Italo-Peruano de Etnomedicina Andina, Lima, Peru, October 27-30, 1993: 21-22.

122. Uchida, S. et al., "Prolongation of Life Span of Stroke-Prone Spontaneously Hypertensive Rats (SHRSP) Ingesting Persimmon Tannin," *Chemical and Pharmaceutical Bulletin* 38 (1990): 1049-1052.

123. Capasso, F., "Medicinal Plants: An Approach to the Study of Naturally Occurring Drugs," *Journal of Ethnopharmacology* 13 (1985): 111-114.

124. Martin, G. J., "Biochemistry of the Bioflavonoids," *Annals of the New York Academy of Sciences* 61 (1955): 646-651.

125. Clementson, C. A. B. and L. Anderson, "Plant Polyphenols as Antioxidants for Ascorbic Acid," *Annals of the New York Academy of Sciences* 136 (1966): 339-378.

126. Middleton, E. and C. Kandaswami, "Plant Flavonoid Modulation of Immune and Inflammatory Cell Functions," David M. Klurfeld, (ed.), *Human Nutrition—A Comprehensive Treatise*, vol. 8: Nutrition and Immunology (New York, NY: Plenum Press, 1993): 239-266.

127. Kühnau, J., "The Flavonoids. A Class of Semi-Essential Food Components: Their Role in Human Nutrition," Geoffrey H. Bourne, (ed.), *World Review of Nutrition and Dietetics* 24 (Basel, Switzerland: S. Karger, 1974): 117-191.

128. Hertog, M. G. L. et al., "Intake of Potentially Anticarcinogenic Flavonoids and Their Determinants in Adults in the Netherlands," *Nutrition and Cancer* 20 (1993): 21-29.

129. Mukhtar, H. et al., "Tea Components: Antimutagenic and Anticarcinogenic Effects," *Preventive Medicine* 21 (1992): 351-360.

130. Brody, J. E., "Scientists Seeking Possible Wonder Drugs in Tea," *The New York Times*, March 14, 1991.

131. Kada, T. et al., "Detection and Chemical Identification of Natural Bio-antimutagens," *Mutation Research* 15 (1985): 127-132.

132. Schneider-Leukel, K. et al., "Flavonoid Release from Herbal Drugs into Medicinal Teas," *Planta Medica* 58, suppl. 1 (1992): A676-A677.

133. Niwa, Y. and Y. Miyachi, "Antioxidant Action of Natural Health Products and Chinese Herbs," *Inflammation* 10 (1986): 79-91.

134. Niwa, Y. et al., "Why are Natural Plant Medicinal Products Effective in Some Patients and not in Others with the Same Disease?" *Planta Medica* 57 (1991): 299-304.

135. Bombardelli, E. and P. Mortazzoni, "*Vitis vinefera* L.," *Fitoterapia* 66 (1995): 291-317.

136. Alpha Chemical and Biomedical Laboratories, Inc., Petaluma, California, November 21, 1995, Report ACBL Job #9151-95.

137. Rizzi, R. et al., "Mutagenic and Antimutagenic Activities of *Uncaria tomentosa* and its Extracts," 1st Colloque European D'Ethnopharmacologie, Metz, France, March 22-24, 1990, abstract.

138. Rizzi, R. et al., "Bacterial Cytotoxicity, Mutagenicity and Antimutagenicity of *Uncaria tomentosa* and its Extracts. Antimutagenic Activity of *Uncaria tomentosa* Bulb in Humans," 1st Colloque European D'Ethnopharmacologie, Metz, France, March 22-24, 1990, abstract.

139. Rizzi, R. et al., "Mutagenic and Antimutagenic Activities of *Uncaria tomentosa* and its Extracts," *Journal of Ethnopharmacology* 38 (1993): 63-77.

140. Cameron, E. and L. Pauling, "Supplemental Ascorbate in the Supportive Treatment of Cancer: Prolongation of Survival Times in Terminal Human Cancer," *Proceedings of the National Academy of Sciences USA* 73 (1976): 3685-3689.

141. Watson, R. R. and T. K. Leonard, "Selenium and Vitamins A, E, and C: Nutrients with Cancer Preventive Properties," *Journal of the American Dietetic Association* 86 (1986): 505-510.

142. Balanehru, S. and B. Nagarajan, "Intervention of Adriamycin Induced Free Radical Damage," *Biochemistry International* 28 (1992): 735-744.

143. Challem, J., "Research Update: Beta Carotene and Radiation Damage; Folic Acid and Colorectal Cancers," *Vitamin Retailer*, April 1994: 40-41.

144. Schimmer, O. and M. Lindenbaum, "Tannins with Antimutagenic Properties in the Herb of *Alchemilla* Species and *Potentilla anserina*," *Planta Medica* 61 (1995): 141-145.

145. Liu, J. and A. Mori, "Antioxidant and Free Radical Scavenging Activities of *Gastrodia elata* Bl. and *Uncaria rynchophylla* (Miq.) Jacks," *Neuropharmacology* 31 (1992): 1287-1298.

146. Aruoma, O. I. et al., "Antioxidant and Pro-oxidant Properties of Active Rosemary Constituents: Carnosol and Carnosic Acid," *Xenobiotica* 22 (1992): 257-268.

147. Balanchru, S. and B. Nagarajan, "Protective Effect of Oleanolic Acid and Ursolic Acid Against Lipid Peroxidation," *Biochemistry International* 24 (1991): 981-990.

148. Larson, R. A., "The Antioxidants of Higher Plants," *Phytochemistry* 27 (1988): 969-978.

149. Brell, Guisella Tesoro and family, personal communication, August 8, 1995.

150. Brell, Guisella Tesoro and family, personal communication, August 7, 1995.

151. Elena Irribarren, personal communication, August 7, 1995.

152. Brell, Arturo, "Nuevos Conceptos Sobre Problemas Degenerativos (El Cancer)," Lima, March 1977, 3 pp.

153. Lancho, Manases Fernandez, personal communication, August 8, 1995.

154. Lancho, Manases Fernandez, Lima, letter to Arturo Brell, May 2, 1964.

155. Luna, Angel, personal communication, August 8, 1995.

156. De Ugaz, Olga Lock, Pontificia Universidad Catolica del Peru, personal communication, August 15, 1995.

157. Balandrin, M. F. et al., "Natural Plant Chemicals: Sources of Industrial and Medicinal Materials," *Science* 228 (June, 1985): 1154-1160.

158. Law, K. H. and N. P. Das, "Studies on the Formation and Growth of *Uncaria elliptica* Tissue Culture," *Journal of Natural Products* 53 (1990): 125-130.

159. "La micropropagación in vitro evitariá extinción genética de la 'uña de gato'," *El Comercio* (Lima), October 23, 1995: A9.

160. De Ugaz, O. L., "Revision del Genero *Uncaria. Uncaria tomentosa* y *Uncaria guianensis*: Las "Uña de Gato," *Revista de Química* 9, no 1 (1995): 49-61.

161. Cabieses, Fernando, Ministry of Health, Lima, personal communication, August 17, 1995.

162. "Krellendorntee aus Peru hilft einem AIDS-Kranken," *Wien Kurier*, April 29, 1987.

163. "Planta que curaría el Sida es la 'uña de gato'," *El Comercio* (Lima), November 29, 1988.

164. Reuters, "AIDS therapy for rich, charities say," *The Globe and Mail*, September 28, 1995, A8.

165. "Heterosexual Transmission Responsible for 75% of World's HIV Cases," *British Journal of Sexual Medicine* 19 (March/April, 1992): 55.

166. Gotuzzo, E. et al., "En Marcha Seria Investigacion: Uña de Gato y Pacientes con el VIH," *De Ciencia y Tecnologia* no. 34 (October, 1993).

167. Inchaustegui Gonzales, Roberto, *Estudio Preliminar Sobre CAS y SIDA Utilizando Plantas Medicinales, Años 1989-1994, Hospital IPSS, Iquitos, Peru* (Iquitos, Peru: Hospital del Instituto Peruano de Seguridad Social Iquitos Comite ETS-SIDA, February 1993), 24 pp.

168. "Médico curó a siete enfermos de Sida con plantas selváticas," *El Comercio* (Lima), February 26, 1994.

169. Santos, Guillermo, letter to Robert Mix, undated; medical interpretation of original report of Dr. Roberto Inchaustegui Gonzales.

170. Uphof, J. C. Th., *Dictionary of Economic Plants* (New York, NY: Second edition, Verlag von J. Cramer, 1968): 188.

171. Schultes, Richard Evans and Robert E. Raffauf, *The Healing Forest, Medicinal and Toxic Plants of the Northwest Amazonia* (Portland, Or: Dioscorides Press, 1990): 86.

172. "Con 'uña de gato' logran éxito en lucha contra SIDA en Austria," *El Comercio* (Lima), July 18, 1993: A1.

173. Levy, J. A., "A New Human Herpesvirus: KSHV or HHV8?," *The Lancet* 34 (September 23, 1995): 786.

174. Whitby, D. et al., "Detection of Kaposi Sarcoma Associated Herpesvirus in Peripheral Blood of HIV-infected Individuals and Progression to Kaposi's Sarcoma," *The Lancet* 34 (September 23, 1995): 799-802.

175. Aquino, R. et al., "Plant Metabolites. Structure and *In Vitro* Antiviral Activity of Quinovic Acid Glycosides from *Uncaria tomentosa* and *Guettarda platypoda*," *Journal of Natural Products* 52 (1989): 679-685.

176. Keplinger, Ursula, "Einfluss von Krallendornextract auf Retrovirale Infektioned," *Zürcher AIDS Kongress*, Zurich, Switzerland, October 16 and 17, 1992, program and abstracts.

177. Keplinger, U. M., "Therapy of HIV-Infected Individuals in the Pathological Categories CDC A1 and CDC B2 with a Preparation Containing IMM-207," *IV. Österreichischer AIDS-Kongress*, Vienna, Austria, September 17 and 18, 1993, abstracts: 45.

178. Urbina, Humberto Ruiz, *Experiencias con el Empleor de la Plants "Uncaria tomentosa" o "Uña de Gato" en Clínica Veterinaria de Perros y Gatos*, Lima, Peru, May, 1994, 11 pp.

179. Fernandez, Victor, Universidad Mayor de San Marcos, Lima, personal communication, August 16, 1995.

180. Urbina, Humberto Ruiz, Profesor Emerito de la Universidad Nacional Mayor de San Marcos, Curriculm Vitae.

181. Urbina, Humberto Ruiz, "Fitoterapia Antitumoral: Plantas con Propiedades Inmunoestimulantes," Lima, Peru, 6 pp., undated.

182. Urbina, Humberto Ruiz, "Usos Medicinales de la Planta Peruana "Uña de Gato," report presented at the "Uña de Gato" First International Congress, Geneva, May 30-31, 1994, 9 pp.

183. Mockett, A. P. A. and M. S. Stahl., "Comparing How Puppies with Passive Immunity Respond to Three Canine Parvovirus Vaccines," *Veterinary Medicine*, May 1995: 430-438.

184. Fries, C. L. and A. M. Remedios, "The Pathogenesis and Diagnosis of Canine Hip Dysplasia: A Review," *Canadian Veterinary Journal* 36 (1995): 494-502.

185. Remedios, A. M. and C. L. Fries, "Treatment of Canine Hip Dysplasia: A Review," *Canadian Veterinary Journal* 36 (1995): 503-509.

186. Shaw, F. P., "FIV: A Quiet Killer," *Cats*, December 1993: 55-56.

187. Staples, K. M., "Fighting Feline Leukemia," *Cat Fancy*, March 1993: 14, 16, 18 and 19.

188. Whitworth, Eugene, letter to Arturo Brell, April 8, 1970.

189. Brell, Guisella Tesoro, personal communication, Lima, August 19, 1995.

190. Whitworth, Eugene, letter to Arturo Brell, May 29, 1971.

191. Press release, Tucson, Arizona, June 1971, "Americans Credited with Finding Herb that Cures Cancer." Note the slant that Whitworth put on the title, reasoning then that no one would take a Peruvian discoverer seriously enough.

192. Brell, Arturo, letter to President Richard Nixon, March 29, 1971.

193. Whitworth, Eugene, letter to Arturo Brell, February 24, 1971.

194. Moss, Ralph W., *Questioning Chemotherapy* (Brooklyn, NY: Equinox Press, 1995): 21.

195. Whitworth, Eugene, letter to Arturo Brell, August 1971, citing letter received from Robert J. Avery, Jr., NCI, dated July 15, 1971.

196. Avery, Robert J., letter to Dr. Anthony Donovan, AID, c/o American Embassy, Lima, Peru, August 17, 1971.

197. Whitworth, Eugene, letter to Arturo Brell, November 15, 1971.

198. Avery, Robert J., U.S. National Institutes of Health, letter to Dr. Anthony Donovan, AID, c/o American Embassy, Lima, Peru, October 26, 1971.

199. Hartwell, Jonathan L., U.S. National Institutes of Health, letter to K. Jewers, September 9, 1974.

200. Jewers, K., Tropical Products Institute, letter to Gael Dohany, October 11, 1974.

201. Dohany, Gael, London, England, letter to Arturo Brell, December 3, 1974.

202. Giribaldi B., Cecilia, letter to Arturo Brell, May 25, 1976.

203. Miranda, Hector J. Vega (ACPC), Lima, letter to the author, October 16, 1995.

204. *Uña de Gato*, Instituto Nacional de Investigación Agraria (INIA), Estación Experimental Pucullpa, Programa Nacional de Investigación en Agroforestería, Pucullpa, Peru, 1995 (brochure).

205. "Desarrollan alternativa para conservar planta, 'Uña de Gato'," *El Comercio* (Lima), August 31, 1995.

206. Brell, Guisella Tesoro, personal communication, October 13, 1995.

207. Napa, Miguel Ventura, Ministerio de Agricultura, Instituto de Recursos Naturales, San Isidro, Lima, Peru, letter to the author, February 17, 1995.

208. Paz y Miño C. G. et al., "Useful Lianas of the Siona-Secoya Indians from Amazonian Ecuador," *Economic Botany* 49 (1995): 269-275.

209. Dobson, Andy, "Biodiversity and Human Health," *Trends in Ecology and Evolution* 10 (October 1995): 390-391.

210. "Desde hace tres años exportan la 'Uña de Gato'," *El Comercio* (Lima), August 1, 1993: A8.

211. "Alemán dice que en la Selva hay plantas que controlarían cáncer," *El Comercio* (Lima), 1971 (date and page number missing).

212. Cantuarias, Oscar Miró-Quesada, Institutos Nacionales de Salud, Lima, letter to Arturo Brell, December 22, 1972.

213. Cisneros, Antonio, "Milagro en la Selva: la Uña de Gato: A Miracle of the Peruvian Jungle," *El Dorado* magazine (Lima), December-February, 1996: 18-21.

214. McSweeney, Daniel, "1995 Industry Survey: Industry Rings Up Solid Sales Gain," *Vitamin Retailer*, December 1995: 30, 35-36, and 38.

215. "Expertos Viajarán a Chernobyl para investigar Tratamiento con 'uña de gato'," *El Comercio* (Lima), December 16, 1995: A18.

216. Belaunde, Meche Garcia, "Que no le den liebre por gato," *El Comercio* (Lima), October 15, 1995: E12.

217. Legon, Jeordan, "Hispanics' use of 'miracle' herb worries the FDA," *The Seattle Times*, December 25, 1995: D2.

218. Plowman, Timothy, "The Ethnobotany of Coca (Erythroxylum spp., Erythroxylaceae)," G. T. Prance and J. A. Kallunki (eds.), *Ethnobotany in the Neotropics*, Proceedings: Ethnobotany in the Neotropics Symposium, Society for Economic Botany, June 13-14, 1993, Oxford, Ohio, *Advances in Economic Botany*, 1 (Bronx, NY: New York Botanical Garden, 1984): 62-111.

219. Lewis, W. and M. P. Elvin-Lewis, "Basic, Quantitative and Experimental Research Phases of Future Ethnobotany with Reference to the Medicinal Plants of South America," G. T. Prance et al. (eds.), *Ethnobotany and the Search for New Drugs*, Symposium on Ethnobotany and the Search for New Drugs, Forteleza, Brazil, November 30 to December 2, 1993, *Ciba Foundation Symposium*, 186 (New York, NY: John Wiley and Sons, 1994): 60-76.

Index